Teen Health

Course 2

Student Activities Workbook

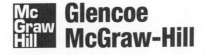 **Glencoe McGraw-Hill**

New York, New York   Columbus, Ohio   Chicago, Illinois   Peoria, Illinois   Woodland Hills, California

Glencoe/McGraw-Hill

A Division of The **McGraw·Hill** *Companies*

Printed in the United States of America.

Send all inquiries to:
Glencoe/McGraw-Hill
21600 Oxnard Street, Suite 500
Woodland Hills, CA 91367

ISBN 0-07-826154-6 (Student Edition)
ISBN 0-07-826155-4 (Teacher Annotated Edition)

5 6 7 8 9   009   06 05 04

Table of Contents

Introduction

This Workbook contains Study Guides, Activities, and Health Inventories to accompany the chapters in your student textbook.

The Study Guides are to be completed as you read each lesson. They will help you check your understanding of lesson content. Each Study Guide consists of approximately 15 items. The items outline the main ideas in the chapter. After you have completed all the items, you can use the Study Guide to review the information in the chapter as a whole.

Following each Study Guide, there are Activities—one for each lesson in your textbook. The Activities give you opportunities to apply your knowledge and practice health-related skills. A variety of formats is offered, including fill-ins, short answer, matching, classifying, and sequencing. In some Activities, you are asked to complete a table after reading a short passage or to label or number items on a diagram. Still other Activities involve writing short paragraphs, essays, or letters.

A Health Inventory follows the Activities for each chapter. Each Health Inventory offers you an opportunity to assess a particular aspect of your health. A typical Health Inventory consists of 15 statements for which you are asked to indicate *yes* if the statement describes you (or *no* if it does not) or to indicate whether the statement describes you *always*, *sometimes*, or *never* (or *always*, *usually*, or *sometimes*). A few of the Health Inventories take the form of checklists in which you are asked to check the items that describe you. The purpose of the Health Inventories is to help you recognize what you are doing that is good for your health and identify behaviors that you need to change.

Chapter 1 Study Guide

STUDY TIPS

✔ Read the chapter objectives.

✔ Look up any unfamiliar words.

✔ Read the questions below before you read the chapter.

   As you read the chapter, answer the following questions. Later you can use this guide to review the information in the chapter.

Lesson 1

1. List four ways to stay physically healthy.

_____

_____

2. List four ways to stay mentally/emotionally healthy.

_____

_____

3. List four ways to stay socially healthy.

_____

_____

4. Define *self-assessment* and relate it to health.

_____

_____

5. Explain the difference between *health* and *wellness*.

_____

_____

Lesson 2

6. Explain how heredity affects one's health.

_____

_____

_____

7. Explain why it is important to your health to know about your physical surroundings.

_____

_____

_____

_____

8. Name three factors, besides heredity and physical surroundings, that influence your health choices.

_____

_____

Lesson 3

9. List six kinds of consequences that might result from taking unnecessary risks.

_____

_____

10. Give an example of cumulative risks and explain why the risks are cumulative.

_____

_____

11. Compare objective thinking with subjective thinking.

_____

_____

12. How is abstinence related to prevention?

_____

_____

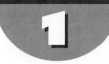

Activity 1   Use with Chapter 1, Lesson 1.

Applying Health Skills

Balancing the Health Triangle

Roy and Karen's health triangles are out of balance. Recommend changes that each could make to balance his or her triangle.

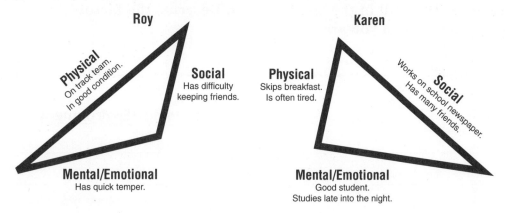

Roy

1. Side of Roy's health triangle I would suggest changing first:

_____

2. Benefit of this change:

_____

3. Other changes Roy could make:

_____

_____

Karen

4. Side of Karen's health triangle I would suggest changing first:

_____

5. Benefits of this change:

_____

6. Other changes Karen could make:

_____

_____

Activity 2 — Applying Health Skills

Put Your Puzzle Together

Think of yourself as a one-of-a-kind jigsaw puzzle. The factors that influence your health are the pieces of the puzzle. What does your puzzle look like? Fill in the blanks below. Describe the factors that make you the person you are.

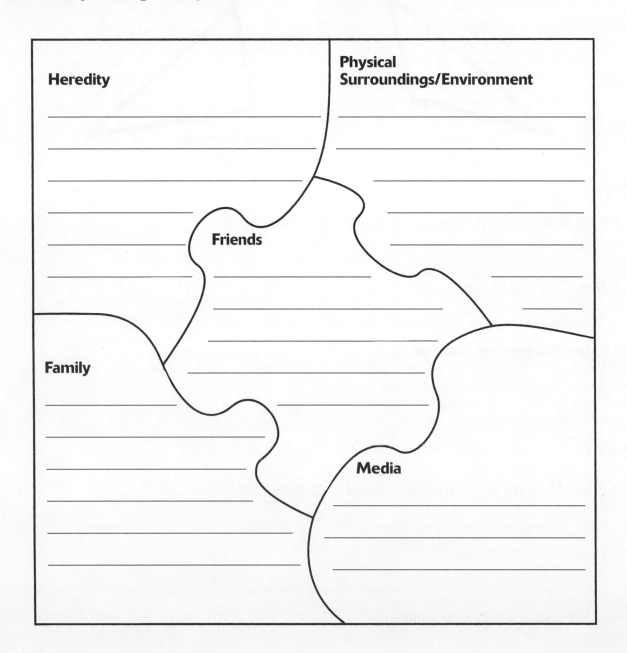

Heredity

_____

_____

_____

_____

Physical Surroundings/Environment

_____

_____

_____

_____

Friends

_____

_____

Family

_____

_____

_____

Media

_____

_____

_____

Activity 3

Applying Health Skills

What's the Risk?

Most activities or actions carry a risk, but all risks are not equal. When there is only a slight chance that something harmful will result from an activity or if the possible harm is minor, the activity can be said to carry a reasonable risk. When there is a good chance that something harmful will result and the possible harm is major, the activity can be said to carry an unreasonable, and unnecessary, risk. Use the chart below to rate the following actions. Write *R* if you think the action is a reasonable risk and *U* if you think the action carries an unreasonable, unnecessary risk. Then replace any unreasonable risk actions with a reasonable action on the line beneath the statement.

Risk Behavior

_____ 1. Sleep fewer than eight hours one night.

_____

_____ 2. Skip breakfast one day.

_____

_____ 3. Lose your temper and pick a fight with a stranger.

_____

_____ 4. Use illegal drugs.

_____

_____ 5. Try a harsh "starvation" diet.

_____

_____ 6. Skip a day of exercising.

_____

_____ 7. Eat mostly high-fat meals.

_____

_____ 8. Skateboard without a helmet.

_____

Chapter 1 Health Inventory

What's Healthy? What's Not?

How well do you understand what it means to be healthy? Read each statement below. Write *true* in the space to the left if you think the statement is true. Write *false* if you think it is false.

_____ 1. The older you become, the more active a role you play in achieving health and wellness.

_____ 2. Your tendency to get some diseases may be hereditary.

_____ 3. It is important to evaluate media messages carefully in order to make healthy choices.

_____ 4. Taking steps to keep something from happening is called *prevention*.

_____ 5. The best way to achieve wellness is to focus on just one part of the health triangle.

_____ 6. Health involves every part of your life.

_____ 7. Your environment may affect your health either positively or negatively.

_____ 8. Physical health is a more important part of wellness than social or mental/emotional health.

_____ 9. Being a truthful and dependable friend can improve your wellness.

_____ 10. Friends, while important, are not a major influence on your health.

_____ 11. There are outside factors, which you cannot control, that affect your health.

_____ 12. A hobby can have a positive effect on your mental/emotional wellness.

_____ 13. Risk behaviors are behaviors that may harm you, but not others.

_____ 14. Your family's cultural background can affect your health.

_____ 15. The key to wellness is to lead a totally trouble-free life and to avoid any potential problems.

Score yourself:

Write the number of questions you answered correctly here.

12–15: Excellent—you know the score on health and wellness.

8–11: Fair—your understanding of health is only moderately healthy.

0–7: Poor—you need to learn more about what it means to be healthy.

Chapter 2 Study Guide

STUDY TIPS
✔ Read the chapter objectives.
✔ Look up any unfamiliar words.
✔ Read the questions below before you read the chapter.

As you read the chapter, answer the following questions. Later you can use this guide to review the information in the chapter.

Lesson 1

1. List the six main health skills.

_____

_____

2. Define stress management.

_____

_____

3. Name two kinds of factors that influence your health choices and give an example of each.

_____

_____

Lesson 2

4. List the sources from which people develop values.

_____

5. Explain the H.E.L.P. criteria.

_____

_____

6. Identify the six steps in the decision-making process.

_____

_____

_____

Lesson 3

7. What are *long-term* and *short-term* goals?

_____

_____

_____

8. What is a goal-setting plan?

_____

_____

9. Identify the five steps of a goal-setting plan.

_____

_____

_____

Lesson 4

10. List the traits that a person who is said to have good character will have.

_____

_____

11. Where do people learn about character?

_____

_____

12. What are some questions that you can ask yourself to learn about your own character?

_____

_____

Activity 4

Use with Chapter 2, Lesson 1.

Applying Health Skills

Practicing Healthful Behaviors

When you practice healthful behaviors, you use skills that protect you from immediate illness or injury and also increase your level of long-term physical wellness. For each of the time periods listed below in column 1, write an example of a healthful behavior that you usually or often do during that period. In column 2, write a new behavior that you could do during that period to help you improve or maintain your health.

Healthful Behaviors That I Practice Daily	New Healthful Behaviors I Can Add
Before School _____ _____ _____	_____ _____ _____
During Classes _____ _____ _____	_____ _____ _____
During Lunch Hour _____ _____ _____	_____ _____ _____
After School _____ _____ _____	_____ _____ _____
In the Evening _____ _____ _____	_____ _____ _____

Activity 5

Applying Health Skills

Have a Decision to Make? Get H.E.L.P.!

Analyze each situation below using the H.E.L.P. criteria. Then, write what you would do in each case.

For each of the situations, answer these questions:	
H (Healthful)	*Is this action healthful?*
E (Ethical)	*Is this action ethical? Does it comform with my values?*
L (Legal)	*Is this action legal?*
P (Parent approval)	*Would my parents approve of this situation?*

1. Leslie wants to rent an R-rated movie. Maura says they're not old enough, but Leslie is sure the video clerk will let her rent it. "We're not babies!" she adds.

What would you do in Maura's place?

H _____

E _____

L _____

P _____

I would . . . _____

2. Steve elbows Martin and points at a woman walking in front of them. A twenty dollar bill has fallen out of her purse. Steve rushes over and picks up the bill, laughing. Martin says that they should return the bill to the woman, but Steve says, "Finders, keepers."

What would you do in Martin's place?

H _____

E _____

L _____

P _____

I would . . . _____

Activity 6
Applying Health Skills

Make a Goal-Setting Plan

Do you have any long-term goals? Then you need a *goal-setting plan*, which identifies a series of steps to take to achieve your goal. In the spaces below, write a goal-setting plan for a long-term goal. Use one of the goals suggested below, or use a goal of your own. Start by writing your goal at the top; then fill in steps you can take on your way to the goal.

Become a doctor	Record a CD	Run a marathon
Start a band	Raise a family	Write a novel

Long-Term Goal

Steps I will take to reach my goal:

_____

_____

Now fill in the blanks below.

To reach my long-term goal, starting tomorrow I should:

_____

_____

The most important short-term goal in my plan is:

_____

_____

Checkpoints I will set to evaluate my progress are:

_____

_____

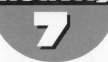

Activity 7

Use with Chapter 2, Lesson 4.

Applying Health Skills

Recognizing Good Character Traits

People who are said to have good character display the following traits: trustworthiness, respect, responsibility, fairness, caring, and citizenship. Read each description of behavior in the boxes below. On the line provided under each box, write the main trait that the person being described is displaying.

---

1. Paolo is an active antismoking supporter. He tries to educate the smokers among his family and friends about the dangers of smoking.

_____

---

4. Philip told his friends that he cannot go to the movies with them as they had planned because he realizes that he needs to study for his math test.

_____

---

2. Andrea is one of the officials for a junior soccer league. Her younger sister is on one of the teams. During the playoffs, although Andrea knew how much winning would mean to her sister, she showed no favoritism in the calls she made as an official.

_____

---

5. When Dennis noticed that Melissa was sitting all alone away from the rest of the class, he went over and sat by her. He smiled and asked her how her day was going.

_____

---

3. Jackie disagrees with practically everything Gwen is saying, but she accepts the fact that Gwen has different opinions.

_____

---

6. When Casey confides in Taylor, Taylor keeps the secret to himself.

_____

Chapter 2 Health Inventory

Taking Responsibility

Read each statement below. Decide whether it describes how you take responsibility for your decisions. Write *always*, *sometimes*, or *never* in the space to the left of each statement.

_____ 1. I seek reliable information before making important decisions.

_____ 2. When making decisions, I recognize which factors are internal and which are external.

_____ 3. I use refusal skills to stand up for my decisions and beliefs.

_____ 4. When making decisions, I carefully consider the consequences of each option.

_____ 5. Before making a decision or taking an action, I think about how it relates to values.

_____ 6. I try to base my decisions on objective knowledge.

_____ 7. I evaluate situations using the H.E.L.P. (Healthful, Ethical, Legal, Parent approval) criteria.

_____ 8. I apply the six-step process when I make decisions.

_____ 9. I am aware that many of the decisions that I make will lead to other decisions.

_____ 10. I use goal-setting plans when making long-term goals.

_____ 11. I use decision making and goal setting to help me get rid of harmful habits.

_____ 12. I try to make decisions that reflect the traits of good character.

_____ 13. When discussing decisions with others, I listen with respect, even if they see situations or ideas differently.

_____ 14. I am willing to accept the consequences of my actions.

_____ 15. I try to make decisions and take actions that help my school and community.

Score yourself:

Give yourself 3 points for each *always* answer, 1 point for each *sometimes*, and 0 for each *never*. Write your score here.

40–45: Excellent—you always take responsibility for your decisions.

30–39: Good—you often take responsibility for your decisions.

19–29: Fair—you can improve your decision-making skills.

Fewer than 19: You need to work on building sound decision-making skills.

Chapter 3 Study Guide

> Study Tips
> ✔ Read the chapter objectives.
> ✔ Look up any unfamiliar words.
> ✔ Read the questions below before you read the chapter.

As you read the chapter, answer the following questions. Later you can use this guide to review the information in the chapter.

Lesson 1

1. Identify the three elements of fitness.

   _____

2. Give two examples of exercises that can help build each of the following: strength, heart and lung endurance, and muscle endurance.

   _____

   _____

   _____

Lesson 2

3. Name five functions of the skeletal system.

   _____

   _____

4. Identify three types of joints.

   _____

   _____

5. Identify the three types of muscle, and give an example of each.

   _____

Lesson 3

6. Explain the difference between pulmonary circulation and systemic circulation.

_____

_____

7. Name the three types of blood vessels. List the four parts of blood.

_____

Lesson 4

8. What are the elements of a good workout?

_____

_____

9. To meet your fitness goals, what three factors should increase over time?

_____

_____

Lesson 5

10. What are the pros and cons of individual and team sports?

_____

_____

_____

_____

11. What effect should playing sports have on your diet?

_____

_____

12. What is *conditioning*, and what are the signs of overtraining?

_____

Activity 8

Applying Health Skills

Dear Dr. Fitness

Imagine that you are a fitness expert. You write a column in a magazine for teens. Your job is to answer letters from readers who have questions about fitness. In today's mail, you received the following two letters asking for advice. Read each letter carefully and write a reply, using facts and ideas from the textbook to deal with each issue.

Letter 1
Dear Dr. Fitness:

By the end of each week, I feel totally drained and tired out. I'm involved in a lot of activities, but most of them are not very physical. For example, I spend a lot of time building models. I think I'm getting enough sleep. Why do I feel tired all the time? What can I do about it?

_____

_____

_____

_____

Letter 2
Dear Dr. Fitness:

I'm not sure what people mean when they talk about aerobic exercise. Which exercises are aerobic? Are they the best types of exercises to do to get fit? I'm kind of new to physical fitness and want to get in shape. What should I do?

_____

_____

_____

_____

_____

_____

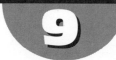

Activity 9

Use with Chapter 3, Lesson 2.

Applying Health Skills

Opposites Attract

Many systems, cycles, and events in nature involve opposites. Simple examples include night and day, young and old, and hot and cold.

Imagine that you are writing articles for an encyclopedia for elementary school students. Apply the idea of opposites to explain the pairs of terms listed below. Using your textbook as a resource, apply the idea of opposites to explain how the terms in a pair relate to each other. Write your explanations on the lines provided. Use language that would be appropriate for elementary school students.

1.
Immovable and Movable Joints

_____
_____
_____
_____
_____

2.
Voluntary and Involuntary Muscles

_____
_____
_____
_____
_____

3.
Contract and Extend

_____
_____
_____
_____

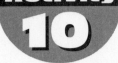 **Activity 10**

Use with Chapter 3, Lesson 3.

Applying Health Skills

Your Circulatory System

The diagram below shows the parts of the circulatory system.
Identify each part by writing its name in the correct box.

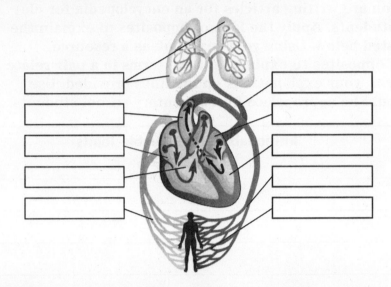

Below is a list of the functions performed by the organs and blood
vessels in the circulatory system. Match each part from the diagram
above to explain the process of circulation in the body. Write the
name of the part in the space provided.

_____ 1. replaces carbon dioxide in blood with oxygen

_____ 2. blood vessel that carries oxygen-rich blood to the heart

_____ 3. chamber that receives oxygen-rich blood from the lungs

_____ 4. chamber that pumps oxygen-rich blood to the aorta

_____ 5. the body's largest artery, which carries blood to branching
arteries

_____ 6. distributes blood away from the heart to all parts of the
body

_____ 7. carry blood to and from body cells

_____ 8. carry low-oxygen blood back to the heart from all parts of
the body

_____ 9. chamber that receives low-oxygen blood in the heart

_____ 10. chamber that sends low-oxygen, high-carbon dioxide blood
out of the heart to the lungs

Activity 11

Use with Chapter 3, Lesson 4.

Applying Health Skills

The Truth About Fitness Programs

Write *true* or *false* next to each statement below.

_____ 1. The first step in setting up a fitness program is to establish a specific goal to inspire you to stick with the program.

_____ 2. A good workout is at least an hour long.

_____ 3. Tight-fitting clothing, such as elasticized body suits, are the best type of clothing to wear when exercising.

_____ 4. If you must exercise outdoors at night, the safest type of clothing includes light colors and reflective coverings.

_____ 5. It is important to choose good exercise equipment.

_____ 6. Wearing sunscreen during a workout is important only if the temperature is high.

_____ 7. If you get injured while engaged in physical activity, treat the injury according to the R.I.C.E. formula.

_____ 8. When planning an exercise program, it is most effective to make a six-month plan and stick to it faithfully.

_____ 9. Every workout should begin with a warm-up, followed by stretching.

_____ 10. Every workout should end with a cool-down, followed by stretching.

_____ 11. The term *intensity* refers to the length of each workout.

_____ 12. For best results, you should gradually increase the frequency of your workouts, while maintaining your intensity at a constant and unchanged level.

_____ 13. When first starting to work out, it is wisest to stay at the lower part of the range of your target heart rate.

_____ 14. Having worked out regularly for two weeks, you should begin to see dramatic results.

_____ 15. It is sometimes necessary to adjust your fitness program or rethink your fitness goals.

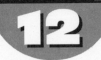

Activity 12 — Use with Chapter 3, Lesson 5.

Applying Health Skills

Sports Facts and Myths

Some of the statements below are facts; others are not. Classify each by writing *fact* or *myth* in the space at the left. On the lines that follow the statements, rewrite the ones you have identified as myths so they are facts.

_____ 1. If you play sports, you may need to take in more calories than a nonathlete.

_____

_____ 2. Foods like bananas, bagels, and fruit juice are good pre-game snacks.

_____

_____ 3. If you drink water while playing sports, you risk getting stomach cramps.

_____

_____ 4. Avoid eating after a game.

_____

_____ 5. Anabolic steroids have many serious side effects.

_____

_____ 6. Different sports demand different levels of strength, endurance, and flexibility.

_____

_____ 7. Feeling sore or tired all the time can be a sign of overtraining.

_____

_____ 8. If you are injured during a game, don't return to the sport until your trainer or doctor says that you are well enough to play.

_____

_____ 9. For wellness and effective conditioning, exercise every day.

_____

Chapter 3 Health Inventory

A Personal Physical Activity and Fitness Profile

Read the statements below. In the space to the left, write *yes* if the statement describes you or *no* if it does not describe you.

_____ 1. I exercise regularly to improve my strength, endurance, and flexibility.

_____ 2. I try not to spend more than half an hour at one time watching television or playing computer games.

_____ 3. For bone growth and strength, I include in my diet foods that are rich in calcium and vitamin D, such as milk.

_____ 4. To build and strengthen muscle tissue, I include protein in my diet food.

_____ 5. I try to sit and stand with correct posture, so that my bones, joints, and muscles maintain proper alignment.

_____ 6. I protect my heart and circulatory system by not smoking.

_____ 7. My fitness program is based on specific, realistic goals, and I feel that these goals help me to stay with the program and to measure my progress.

_____ 8. I take precautions to ensure that I work out safely.

_____ 9. I am careful to do warm-up and stretching exercises before my workouts, as well as cool-down and further stretching exercises after my workouts.

_____ 10. When I get injured playing sports, I always check with a coach, trainer, or doctor before continuing to play.

_____ 11. To guard against sports injuries, I wear appropriate protective equipment, including helmets and pads.

_____ 12. I drink plenty of fluids when I play a sport.

_____ 13. I do not use anabolic steroids.

_____ 14. When I train, I select a variety of activities.

_____ 15. When I train, I take at least one day off a week to give my body a chance to heal.

Score yourself:

Write the number of *yes* answers here.

12–15: You are well-informed about physical activity and fitness and are probably following an effective fitness program.

8–11: You may need to improve your knowledge and practice of safe and effective ways to exercise and keep fit.

Fewer than 8: You need to learn more about physical activity and fitness.

Chapter 4 Study Guide

As you read the chapter, answer the following questions. Later you can use this guide to review the information in the chapter.

Lesson 1

1. Define *nutrients*.

_____

_____

_____

2. List the six major categories of nutrients. Give two examples of food sources for each.

_____

_____

_____

_____

3. Why does the body need fiber?

_____

_____

_____

4. Why should you limit fats, sugar, and salt in your diet?

_____

_____

_____

_____

Lesson 2

5. List the five major food groups shown in the Food Guide Pyramid. After each, list the recommended daily servings for that group.

_____

_____

_____

Lesson 3

6. Why is breakfast such an important meal?

_____

_____

_____

7. What foods are _nutrient dense?_

_____

_____

Lesson 4

8. Define _digestion._ Where does most of the digestive process take place?

_____

_____

_____

9. What is the excretory system? Name the major organs in this system.

_____

_____

_____

Lesson 5

10. What are five factors that determine your healthy weight?

_____

_____

Activity 13 — Applying Health Skills

Name That Nutrient

Write the correct nutrient from the list in the box on each numbered answer line.

Carbohydrates	Minerals	Vitamins
Fats	Proteins	Water

1. _____

- two types: water-soluble and fat-soluble
- help regulate the body's functions
- found in fruits, vegetables, and whole-grain and enriched breads and cereals

2. _____

- supply energy, keep the skin healthy, promote normal growth
- two types: saturated and unsaturated
- found in butter, stick margarine, meat, poultry, dairy products, vegetable oils, nuts, olives, and avocados

3. _____

- include starches and sugars
- provide energy
- found in rice, pasta, breads, potatoes, beans, corn, sugars

4. _____

- helps with digestion and removes wastes
- carries nutrients throughout the body
- regulates body temperature
- found in drinking water

5. _____

- made up of amino acids
- repair body cells and tissues
- found in meat, dairy products, eggs, beans, nuts, and grains

6. _____

- strengthen bones and teeth
- help keep blood healthy
- found in milk, meat, leafy green vegetables, fruits, dry beans, and salt

Activity 14

Use with Chapter 4, Lesson 2.

Applying Health Skills

Let the Pyramid Be Your Guide

The Food Guide Pyramid can help you make daily food choices. Look at the Pyramid; then look at the menus listed beneath it. Beside the food items on each menu, write the letter of the part of the Food Guide Pyramid where that food can be found. Then answer the questions on the next page.

FOOD GUIDE PYRAMID

The Food Guide Pyramid

A Guide to Daily Food Choices

Key

◻ **Fat** (naturally occuring and added)

▽ **Sugars** (added)

These symbols show fats, oils, and added sugars in foods

Fats, Oils, & Sweets
USE SPARINGLY

Milk, Yogurt, & Cheese Group
2–3 Servings

Meat, Poultry, Fish, Dry Beans Eggs, & Nuts Group
2–3 Servings

Vegetable Group
3–5 Servings

Fruit Group
2–4 Servings

Bread, Cereal, Rice, & Pasta Group
6–11 Servings

Poonam's Breakfast

_____ bowl of cereal

_____ milk

_____ glass of orange juice

_____ sliced banana

John's Lunch

_____ bag of chips

_____ two slices of bread

_____ slice of ham

_____ candy bar

_____ can of soda

Meryl's Lunch

_____ licorice whip

_____ candy bar

_____ diet cola

Fred's Dinner

_____ slice of meat loaf

_____ ½ cup of rice

_____ butter

_____ peas

_____ chocolate cake

1. Which is the only meal that included nothing from the tip of the Pyramid?

_____

_____

2. Which meal would you say came closest to the Pyramid's recommendations? Which one was next closest? Explain.

_____

_____

_____

3. Meryl got her lunch from a vending machine. Would you say that it is easy or difficult to follow the Pyramid if you get food from a vending machine? Explain.

_____

_____

_____

Activity 15 — Applying Health Skills

Healthful Choices

Below are the food choices that two teens made over the course of a day. Put a check (✔) next to each choice that is healthful. Then answer the questions on the next page.

Paul's Food Choices

Breakfast

_____ frosted toaster pastry

_____ can of soda

Lunch

_____ two slices of pizza

_____ apple

_____ can of soda

After-School Snack

_____ slice of cake

_____ can of soda

Dinner

_____ spaghetti with tomato sauce

_____ heavily buttered garlic bread

_____ cheese curls

_____ can of soda

_____ slice of cake

Evening Snack

_____ buttered popcorn

_____ can of soda

_____ **Total healthful choices**

Fran's Food Choices

Breakfast

_____ nothing

Lunch

_____ tuna sandwich

_____ orange

_____ low-fat pretzels

_____ carton of fruit juice

After-School Snack

_____ bowl of fruit salad

Dinner

_____ taco salad

_____ salsa

_____ beans

_____ pineapple

Evening Snack

_____ bunch of grapes

_____ **Total healthful choices**

1. Who made the most nutritious food choices on this day?

_____

2. Name one more healthful choice Fran could have made.

_____

3. For which of Paul's meals did he make the most healthful choices?

_____

4. Who had the greater variety of foods in his or her meals?

_____

5. If you could give Paul just *one* piece of advice for improving his food choices, what would it be?

_____

_____

6. Which teen's food choices are most like yours?

_____

_____

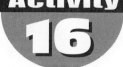

Applying Health Skills

The Digestive Journey

Follow a piece of food from the start to the finish of the digestive system. Fill in each blank with the letter next to the proper term in the right column.

1. The food is torn and ground into small shreds or chunks by the _____.

2. While food is still in the mouth, enzymes in the _____ begin the chemical breakdown of carbohydrates.

3. After it is swallowed, the food enters the _____.

4. The food is pushed along until it reaches the _____, which churns it and mixes it with gastric juice for up to four hours.

5. Next, the food moves into a coiled tube, about 20 feet long, called the _____.

6. Here, the food is further broken down by bile, which is produced in the body's largest gland, the _____.

7. While in the 20-foot tube, nutrients from the digested material pass through the _____ to begin their journey to body cells.

8. After digestion, the body gets rid of waste materials in a process called _____.

9. _____ are a pair of organs that filter water and waste materials from blood.

10. The pouch in which urine is stored in your body is the _____.

11. From there, liquid wastes leave your body through a tube called the _____.

12. Solid wastes are stored in a tube called the _____.

a. villi

b. bladder

c. esophagus

d. excretion

e. kidneys

f. colon

g. liver

h. saliva

i. small intestine

j. stomach

k. teeth

l. urethra

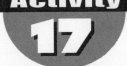 **Activity 17**

Applying Health Skills

Weight Management

Imagine that you are on a quiz show. One of the categories is weight management. The quiz show host presents an answer. You must supply the question.

1. **Answer:** Height, age, gender, inherited body type, and growth pattern

   Question: _____

2. **Answer:** A way to assess body size, taking height and weight into account

   Question: _____

3. **Answer:** Strains the muscles and bones and makes the heart work harder

   Question: _____

4. **Answer:** Fatigue, sleeplessness, and irritability

   Question: _____

5. **Answer:** Heart disease, stroke, and diabetes

   Question: _____

6. **Answer:** About 20 minutes

   Question: _____

7. **Answer:** They are converted into body fat

   Question: _____

8. **Answer:** An eating disorder in which a person repeatedly eats large amounts of food at one time

   Question: _____

9. **Answer:** An eating disorder in which a person has an intense fear of weight gain and starves herself or himself

   Question: _____

10. **Answer:** An eating disorder in which a person repeatedly eats large amounts of food and then purges

    Question: _____

Chapter 4 Health Inventory

Making Nutritious Choices

Read the statements below. In the space at the left, write *yes* **if the statement describes you or** *no* **if it does not describe you.**

_____ **1.** I eat regular meals.

_____ **2.** I drink eight to ten glasses of water a day.

_____ **3.** I participate in moderate physical activity most days of the week.

_____ **4.** I use the Nutrition Facts panels on packaged foods to help me make food choices.

_____ **5.** No more than 30 percent of my daily calories come from fat.

_____ **6.** I eat foods high in fiber each day.

_____ **7.** I eat a variety of foods.

_____ **8.** I eat three to five servings of vegetables each day.

_____ **9.** I eat six to 11 servings of bread, cereal, rice, or pasta each day.

_____ **10.** I eat breakfast each day, usually choosing foods high in complex carbohydrates.

_____ **11.** I choose snack foods that are nutrient dense.

_____ **12.** I eat two to three servings of milk, yogurt, or cheese each day.

_____ **13.** I try to stay within a weight range that is healthy for me.

_____ **14.** I limit the amount of foods I eat that are not nutrient dense.

_____ **15.** I manage my weight in a healthful way.

Score yourself:

How many *yes* answers did you have? Write that number here.

12–15: Excellent

8–11: Good

5–7: Fair

Fewer than 5: Read Chapter 4 carefully to see how you can make better nutrition and weight management choices.

Chapter **5** Study Guide

STUDY TIPS

✔ Read the chapter objectives.

✔ Look up any unfamiliar words.

✔ Read the questions below before you read the chapter.

As you read the chapter, answer the following questions. Later you can use this guide to review the information in the chapter.

Lesson 1

1. Explain the process of tooth decay.

_____

_____

_____

2. List the three layers of the skin.

_____

3. Explain what fingernails, toenails, and hair have in common.

_____

Lesson 2

4. List the parts of the eye.

_____

5. How does the ear work?

_____

_____

_____

Lesson 3

6. Who is a *consumer?*

_____

7. What are *informational* and *image* advertisements?

_____

_____

Lesson 4

8. What is comparison shopping?

_____

_____

9. What are seven kinds of important product information that labels can provide?

_____

_____

Lesson 5

10. Compare the terms commonly known by these acronyms: HMO, PPO, POS.

_____

_____

_____

_____

_____

11. What role do federal, state, and local governments play in health care?

_____

_____

_____

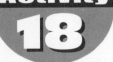

Applying Health Skills

Teeth, Skin, Hair, and Nails

Identify each term in the column on the right by matching it with the proper description in the column on the left. Write the letter of the term in the space to the left of the description.

Descriptions

_____ 1. Tissue containing a tooth's nerve endings and blood vessels.

_____ 2. The substance that gives skin its color.

_____ 3. Do this daily to remove bacteria and excess oils.

_____ 4. A thin, sticky film that builds up on teeth and contributes to tooth decay.

_____ 5. The body's largest organ.

_____ 6. The thin, skinlike layer at the base of each nail.

_____ 7. Contains blood vessels, nerve endings, hair follicles, sweat glands, and oil glands.

_____ 8. Use this to remove trapped food from between teeth.

_____ 9. Tiny openings in the skin.

_____ 10. A hole caused by an acid formed from sugar and plaque.

Terms

a. plaque

b. cuticle

c. dental floss

d. melanin

e. bathe or shower

f. dermis

g. pulp

h. skin

i. cavity

j. pores

Answer the following questions about teeth, skin, hair, and nails. Write your answers on the lines provided.

11. Why is it important to use a toothpaste containing fluoride?

_____

12. What should you do if you have acne?

_____

13. Is washing hair every day the best way to prevent head lice? Explain your answer.

_____

Activity 19 Applying Health Skills

Your Eyes and Ears

Fill in the blanks with the proper terms from below. Then answer questions 13 and 14.

auditory nerve	cochlea	cornea	eardrum
external auditory canal	iris	lens	optic nerve
inner ear	pupil	retina	stirrup

From Light to Sight: The Eye

1. Light enters your eye through the _____.

2. After entering the eye, light passes through an opening called the _____.

3. The size of the opening is determined by the colored portion of the eye, called the _____.

4. The _____ focuses light on the light-sensing part of the inner eye.

5. This light-sensing part of the eye is called the _____.

6. The _____ is a bundle of nerve fibers that send messages to the brain, which interprets them.

From Sound to Hearing: The Ear

7. Sound waves enter the outer ear through the _____.

8. In the middle ear, sound waves make the _____ vibrate.

9. These vibrations move the hammer, the anvil, and the _____.

10. These bones carry the vibrations to the _____.

11. In the inner ear, the vibrations cause fluid in the _____ to move.

12. Tiny hair cells vibrate in the fluid, sending electrical messages to the _____, which relays these signals to the brain, which identifies the sound.

Eye Care and Ear Care

13. To care for your eyes, sit at least _____ feet from the TV set.

14. Normal conversation is about _____ decibels.

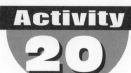

Activity 20 Applying Health Skills

Understanding Ads

Advertisers rely on the following techniques to convince consumers to buy their products: Bandwagon, Beautiful People, Good Times, Status, and Symbols. Each technique has a hidden message. Read the following descriptions and decide which technique the ad uses. Then explain the hidden message behind the ad.

Ad 1
A magazine ad shows a beautiful, smiling young woman with clear skin. The ad reads: "It's a fact . . . nine out of ten supermodels choose Derma-Clear cleansing cream."

1. Technique: _____

2. Hidden Message: _____

Ad 2
This commercial shows a group of hip-looking teens doing a series of dangerous-looking tricks on skateboards. Afterward, they drink some soda. "Dyna-Pop . . . it's extreme!" an announcer says, as loud rock music plays.

3. Technique: _____

4. Hidden Message: _____

Ad 3
In this TV commercial, a very healthy-looking older man holds up a box of cereal. "Bran Nuggets are the smart start to a great day," he says. "Smart folks eat Bran Nuggets for the nutrition they provide. Shouldn't you?"

5. Technique: _____

6. Hidden message: _____

Ad 4
A beloved cartoon character appears in a cereal commercial saying how she eats it several times a day.

7. Technique: _____

8. Hidden Message: _____

Ad 5
A teen girl, surrounded by three teen boys, tells an audience that everyone will like you if you use Sweet Breath mouthwash.

9. Technique: _____

10. Hidden Message: _____

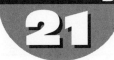

Use with Chapter 5 Lesson 4.

Applying Health Skills

Read the Label

Product labels can tell you a great deal. Look at the labels on these two bottles of shampoo. Use the label information to answer the questions.

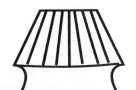

SUDZ SHAMPOO

15 Fluid Ounces

Fights Dandruff!

Directions: Wet hair. Massage into scalp. Rinse. Repeat if desired. For best results, use at least twice a week.

Warning! Avoid contact with eyes. Keep this and all drugs out of the reach of children.

Questions? Comments? Call 1-516-555-5910

$4.95

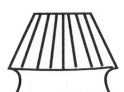

Silky Clean

8.5 Fluid Ounces

Repair Damaged or Stressed Hair

Directions: Apply to wet hair, lather, and rinse. Repeat. For best results, towel-dry hair. Use at least three times a week.

Caution: AVOID CONTACT WITH EYES

Questions? Call 1-800-GO-SILKY

$2.55

1. Jeremy is concerned about dandruff. Which shampoo should he choose?

   _____

2. Susan has a six-year-old brother. Which shampoo requires careful storage?

   _____

3. Phillippa loves the blow-dried look, but has dandruff and brittle hair. Which shampoo would you recommend to her? Why?

   _____

   _____

4. Which shampoo do you suspect has better customer service? Explain.

_____

_____

_____

_____

_____

5. Which shampoo is a better deal? Explain.

_____

_____

_____

_____

_____

6. Which bottle of shampoo will last longer? Explain.

_____

_____

_____

_____

_____

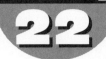

Activity 22

Applying Health Skills

The Health Care System

The health care system is a collection of people and institutions that work together to help people remain healthy and to treat them when they are injured or sick. Identify the parts of the health care system by writing the correct number next to each part listed below.

Health Care System
Goal: Good health for as many people as possible
1. Primary care provider
2. Medical specialist
3. Health care facilities
4. Private health care plan
5. Government health care program

_____ **a.** health departments

_____ **b.** dermatologist

_____ **c.** HMO

_____ **d.** family physician

_____ **e.** allergist

_____ **f.** nursing home

_____ **g.** ophthalmologist

_____ **h.** point-of-service plan

_____ **i.** drug treatment center

_____ **j.** hospice

_____ **k.** nurse practitioner

_____ **l.** PPO

_____ **m.** orthodontist

_____ **n.** health-related information for residents

Imagine that you are explaining to younger students the roles of federal, state, and local governments in health care. Write your explanation on the lines below.

_____

_____

_____

Chapter 5 Health Inventory

Being Smart About Personal Health Care

Read the statements below. In the space at the left, write *yes* if the statement describes you, or *no* if it does not describe you.

_____ 1. I use dental floss at least once a day.

_____ 2. I never clean the inside of my ear canal with a cotton swab.

_____ 3. I sit a least 6 feet from the set when I watch television.

_____ 4. I read the labels of personal-care products before I buy them.

_____ 5. I visit a dentist or dental clinic at least twice a year.

_____ 6. I take a bath or shower every day.

_____ 7. I try not to be out in the sunshine between 10:00 a.m. and 4:00 p.m.

_____ 8. I brush my hair every day.

_____ 9. I do not share my combs, brushes, or hats with other people.

_____ 10. On cold days I wear a hat or earmuffs to cover my ears.

_____ 11. If I have acne, I keep the area clean and keep my hands off the blemishes.

_____ 12. I recognize my personal needs and wants.

_____ 13. I know that advertising claims that seem to be too good to be true usually are.

_____ 14. I compare unit prices when making purchasing decisions.

_____ 15. I brush my teeth at least twice a day.

Score yourself:

How many *yes* answers did you have? Write that number here.

12–15: Excellent—you know the score on being a smart and healthy consumer.

8–11: Good—your understanding of how to be a smart health care consumer is moderate.

5–7: Fair—you need to learn more about being a smart health care consumer.

Fewer than 5: Read Chapter 5 carefully to see how you can improve your health care consumer habits.

Chapter 6 Study Guide

As you read the chapter, answer the following questions. Later you can use this guide to review the information in the chapter.

Lesson 1

1. What are *hormones?*

_____

_____

2. What is the function of the endocrine system? What glands form the system?

_____

_____

3. What is metabolism? What gland produces the hormone that regulates it?

_____

_____

4. Define *puberty.*

_____

Lesson 2

5. What is the *reproductive system?*

_____

_____

6. List the parts of the male reproductive system.

Lesson 3

7. What is *fertilization?*

8. Define *menstruation.*

9. List the parts of the female reproductive system.

Lesson 4

10. Describe how the body is organized, from cells to body systems.

11. What structures within cells influence heredity? Define the structures.

Lesson 5

12. List the stages of life.

13. Name three substances you should protect yourself from.

Activity 23

Applying Health Skills

The Endocrine System

Identify each gland described below by writing its name on the line provided.

_____ 1. Produces several hormones that control the work of other glands and organs. It also regulates the body's growth and development.

_____ 2. Located behind the stomach, this gland controls the level of sugar in the blood and provides the small intestine with digestive chemicals.

_____ 3. These glands produce hormones that control the body's response to emergencies and excitement.

_____ 4. Located alongside the windpipe, this gland regulates body growth and the rate of metabolism.

_____ 5. These are the female reproductive glands.

_____ 6. These small glands are found inside another gland in the endocrine system. They regulate the levels of calcium and phosphorus in the blood.

_____ 7. These are the male reproductive glands.

Read each situation described below. Identify which type of change best describes each teen's experience by writing *P* for physical changes, *M* for mental growth, *E* for emotional changes, and *S* for social development.

_____ 1. Yesterday Sandy was feeling great about life. Then she got a C on a science test for which she had studied very hard. This morning Sandy feels so gloomy that she doesn't want to get out of bed.

_____ 2. Bart and his friends often go to the movies. The boys have seen almost every superhero movie made. Today, Bart wants to see something different. His friends see a superhero movie, while Bart sees a comedy.

_____ 3. Sandra listens while her friends argue over which musical artist is best. They ask Sandra for her opinion. Sandra says that she likes one performer better but agrees that the other one might appeal more to some people.

_____ 4. Mitch goes to a family reunion, where he hardly says a word. He's afraid that his cousins will tease him, since his voice has been cracking and squeaking a lot lately.

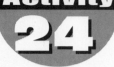

Activity 24

Applying Health Skills

The Male Reproductive System

Some of the statements below are true; others are false. Classify each statement by writing *true* or *false* in the space at the left. On the lines that follow the statements, rewrite the false ones to make them true.

_____ 1. Sperm are first produced shortly before puberty begins.

_____

_____ 2. Testosterone is produced by the prostate gland.

_____

_____ 3. The muscular action that forces semen through the urethra and out of the penis is called ejaculation.

_____

_____ 4. Sterility can be caused by smoking and by certain diseases but not by exposure to environmental hazards.

_____

_____

_____ 5. Males should always wear protective gear when participating in contact sports to help prevent injuries to the reproductive organs.

_____

_____ 6. The urethra is a small tube that runs from the testes along the length of the penis.

_____

_____ 7. Sperm are stored in a network of tubes called the epididymis, located behind the testes.

_____

_____ 8. Testicular cancer is rare, but it is the most common cancer in American males between the ages of 55 and 70.

_____

_____ 9. Semen is a mixture of sperm and fluids.

_____

Activity 25 · Applying Health Skills

Caring for the Female Reproductive System

Below is a list of problems of the female reproductive system. Complete the chart by filling in the cause, symptoms, and treatment or preventive measures for each problem.

Problem	Cause	Symptoms	Treatment or Preventive Measures
1. Vaginitis			
2. Premenstrual syndrome (PMS)			
3. Toxic Shock Syndrome (TSS)			
4. Infertility			

Answer the questions below and on the next page about the female reproductive system. Write your answers on the lines provided.

5. What are the four main functions of the female reproductive system?

_____

_____

_____

_____

6. Explain the function of the fallopian tubes.

_____

_____

_____

7. List four events during the menstrual cycle.

_____

_____

_____

_____

8. List three ways to care for the female reproductive system.

_____

_____

_____

_____

Activity 26

Applying Health Skills

From Cell to Self

Complete the following paragraphs. Write the correct term listed below in each space.

pregnancy	body systems	cells	chromosomes	embryo
fertilization	fetus	genes	organs	tissues

The tiny building blocks of your body are called (1) _____. At one time, you were a single cell formed as a result of (2) _____. (3)_____ generally lasts a little over nine months. Your development may have taken a little more or a little less time. Your first stage of development, lasting about eight weeks, was as an (4) _____. From then until your birth, you were a (5) _____.

As you developed within your mother's womb, your cells developed into (6) _____, which are groups of similar cells that do a particular job. You also developed (7) _____, body parts made up of different tissues joined together to perform a function. Groups of organs that work together to carry out related tasks formed your (8) _____, such as your digestive, endocrine, and reproductive systems.

Each cell in your body contains (9) _____, threadlike structures that carry the codes for traits you inherited from your parents. You inherited (10) _____ for each trait from each parent. These genes react in complex ways, resulting in your particular set of inherited characteristics.

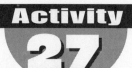

Activity 27

Use with Chapter 6, Lesson 5.

Applying Health Skills

It's a Wonderful Life

Read the list below, which describes developmental events in a person's life. Then write the letters of the events under the corresponding life stage.

Events	Life Stages
a. George begins a career.	**Infancy**
b. George's interactions with his friends become more and more important to him.	1. _____
	2. _____
c. George learns to walk and talk.	**Toddler**
d. George begins to take on greater responsibility.	3. _____
e. George begins to enjoy complex and challenging games.	4. _____
f. The personality that George will have as an adult begins to take shape.	**Preschooler**
	5. _____
g. George's weight triples.	6. _____
h. George likes to imitate his siblings and parents.	**Late Childhood**
	7. _____
i. George works to understand the meaning of his life.	8. _____
j. George learns to sit up.	**Adolescence**
k. George uses the toilet for the first time.	9. _____
	10. _____
l. George's favorite activities are singing and making up elaborate stories.	**Adulthood**
	11. _____
	12. _____

Chapter **6** Health Inventory

Growing and Developing

Read the statements below. In the space to the left of each, write *yes* if the statement describes you, or *no* if it does not describe you.

_____   1. I take a daily bath or shower.

_____   2. I am learning to express my emotions healthfully.

_____   3. I believe that pregnant women should avoid alcohol, tobacco, and other drugs.

_____   4. I have regular physical checkups.

_____   5. I am developing a sense of who I am.

_____   6. I know that males should examine their testes once a month and that females should examine their breasts once a month.

_____   7. I am learning to accept my body and its characteristics.

_____   8. I try to face feelings of anger, sadness, or frustration instead of hiding them.

_____   9. I accept the rate at which my body is developing.

_____   10. I am ready to accept responsibility for my actions.

_____   11. I recognize that each stage of life holds challenges and rewards.

_____   12. I realize that mood swings are a normal part of adolescence.

_____   13. I believe that my teen years will serve as a bridge from childhood to adulthood.

_____   14. When I have a disagreement with others, I can discuss the problem calmly.

_____   15. I am not afraid to have my own personal views.

Score yourself:

Write the number of *yes* answers here.

12–15: Excellent

8–11: Good

Fewer than 8: You are going through a period of growth and development. Think about how you can better prepare yourself for the exciting years ahead.

Chapter 7 Study Guide

As you read the chapter, answer the following questions. Later you can use this guide to review the information in the chapter.

Lesson 1

1. Identify the signs of good mental and emotional health.

_____

_____

_____

2. What are the three most important factors that shape your personality? Over which of these do you have control?

_____

3. Explain the difference between *self-concept* and *self-esteem*.

_____

_____

Lesson 2

4. What are some suggestions for effectively managing fear and effectively managing anger?

_____

_____

_____

5. List four of the emotional or physical reactions involved in the grieving process.

_____

_____

Lesson 3

6. Discuss the difference between *distress* and *eustress*.

_____

_____

7. Explain how the body responds to stress.

_____

_____

Lesson 4

8. Explain the difference between *anxiety disorders* and *mood disorders*.

_____

_____

_____

_____

9. Define *depression*.

_____

_____

_____

_____

10. Explain how you can help a suicidal friend.

_____

_____

_____

Activity 28 **Applying Health Skills**

Good Mental and Emotional Health Traits

Read each statement below. Then decide which qualities of good mental and emotional health the speaker could use to improve his or her outlook. Write the letter of the appropriate quality in the space at the left. Then rewrite the statement to reflect that quality.

_____ 1. "This pitcher is too good for me. I know I'll strike out."

_____

_____ 2. "I don't like my new neighbors. They dress in weird clothes."

_____

_____ 3. "Shut up! I've had a rotten day, and the last thing I need to put up with is a whiny little brother."

_____

_____ 4. "I'm going to make straight A's even if it means studying five hours a day."

_____

_____ 5. "I'm not going to try out. I tried out last time and didn't make it. I'm no good at it, anyway."

_____

_____ 6. "Who are you to tell me how to draw? I think your sketch is dumb."

_____

Mental and Emotional Qualities

a. Have a positive attitude and outlook on life.

b. Accept your limitations and set realistic goals.

c. Have a positive view of yourself and others.

d. Be resilient, able to bounce back from a disappointment, difficulty, or crisis.

e. Act responsibly at school, at home, and in social situations.

f. Be aware of your feelings and be able to express those feelings in healthy ways.

g. Accept constructive feedback without becoming angry.

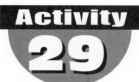

Activity 29   Use with Chapter 7, Lesson 2.

Applying Health Skills

Dealing with Emotions

Read each situation and answer the questions that follow.

1. Rob has been having a string of disappointments. He did not qualify for the marching band and his two best friends did. He tries hard, but his Spanish class is becoming more and more of a mystery. Then after weeks of worry, Rob finally got up the nerve to ask Nancy to the school dance. She turned him down. Each of these developments has aroused strong emotions in Rob. *What emotion might each of the incidents have triggered in Rob?*

_____

_____

2. Felicia is very angry with Harriet. Felicia feels that when she, Harriet, and their friends are together, Harriet seems to contradict everything that Felicia tries to say. Felicia feels that there is nothing that she can say without Harriet attacking it. The more Felicia thinks about it, the angrier she gets with Harriet. *How should Felicia deal with these emotions?*

_____

3. Timmy's mother is going to get married. His new stepdad has two children who are a little older than Timmy. At the end of the school term, Timmy and his mother will be moving out of state to join his new family. Although Timmy is excited about the move, he is sad to leave his friends and old school. He is also a little frightened, although he really doesn't know why. He thinks that he has so many different emotions all tangled together that he doesn't know how he feels. *How do you suggest that Timmy deal with these emotions?*

_____

4. Maura and Cindy both worked hard to try out for the school play and each of them did her best. When the parts were posted, neither of them had made the cast. Both of them felt very disappointed. Maura burst into tears and ran to find a friend to talk to. Cindy quietly walked away to be alone. *What might each girl's way of dealing with the emotion of disappointment reveal?*

_____

5. Claudia has been upset for weeks. She has become irritable with just about everyone. Eating has become one of her few comforts. She turns to food more and more often. Today, after school, she was invited to go to a beer party. "Why not," said Claudia, "I need to blow off steam." *What are three positive alternative activities that could replace the risk behaviors Claudia is using to deal with her emotions?*

Activity 30 — Applying Health Skills

Manage Your Top Stressors

Major events can cause negative stress. So can everyday irritations. Write your top three stressors, listing them from most to least stressful. (Choose from the list or think of your own.) For each of your stressors, list a coping skill to help you manage stress. After each skill, write a plan for using that skill the next time you face that stressor.

Common Stressors

- trouble with teacher or principal
- personal health problems
- arguing with parents
- arguing with brother or sister
- getting glasses or braces
- worrying about appearance
- meeting new people
- illness of a family member
- death of a pet
- end of a close friendship

My Top 3 Stressors

1. _____

2. _____

3. _____

Coping Skills for Managing Stress

- stay healthy
- be physically active
- relax
- manage your time
- maintain a positive outlook
- talk

1. Coping Skill: _____

   Plan: _____

2. Coping Skill: _____

   Plan: _____

3. Coping Skill: _____

   Plan: _____

Activity 31 — Applying Health Skills

Dealing with Mental Disorders

Read each situation. Then answer the questions below and on the next page.

Situation 1

Mark is very close to his older brother Stan. When Stan left for college, Mark felt sad. Everyone assumed that Mark would get used to Stan being gone, but he hasn't. It has been almost three months now. Everything seems hopeless and pointless to Mark. He often goes straight home after school. When his friends invite him to join them, he always shrugs his shoulders and shakes his head no.

1. What type of mental and emotional problem do Mark's symptoms point to?

_____

2. What specific disorder might Mark have?

_____

3. What would you do if you were Mark's friend?

_____

_____

Situation 2

Celia has always been a little shy. Moving to a new school didn't help. Celia is often absent. When she comes to school, she doesn't really talk to anyone except the two friends she has made in her new neighborhood. Even they notice that she is very tense at school. They know that she can sing very well because they have heard her. However, when they suggest that she try out for choir, her face turns red. She says she just couldn't sing with all those people. She can't even face the people at school.

4. What type of mental and emotional problem might Celia's behavior indicate?

_____

5. What specific disorder might Celia have?

_____

6. What could you suggest to Celia's friends?

_____

_____

_____

Situation 3

Frank has been sad ever since his parents divorced. He used to belong to the band, but he didn't bother to try out this year. He spends all of his free time alone in his room with the door locked. The other day Frank gave his CD collection to his best friend.

7. What might Frank's behavior suggest?

_____

8. Do you think Frank can handle this problem alone?

_____

_____

9. What would you do if you were Frank's friend and he did not seek help?

_____

Chapter 7 Health Inventory

Your Mental and Emotional Health

Read the statements below. In the space at the left, write *yes* if the statement describes you or *no* if it does not describe you.

_____ **1.** I have a positive attitude and outlook on life.

_____ **2.** I accept my limitations and set realistic goals.

_____ **3.** I have a positive view of myself and others.

_____ **4.** I am resilient.

_____ **5.** I act responsibly at school, at home, and in social situations.

_____ **6.** I am aware of my feelings and express them in healthy ways.

_____ **7.** I accept constructive feedback without getting angry.

_____ **8.** I ask for help when I need it.

_____ **9.** I focus on my strengths and work to develop new skills.

_____ **10.** I respect others with their differences and similarities.

_____ **11.** I'm willing to try new things.

_____ **12.** I am developing coping skills to manage stress.

_____ **13.** I know the signs of mental and emotional problems.

_____ **14.** I know where students in my school can get help for mental and emotional problems.

_____ **15.** I understand and accept myself.

Score yourself:

Write the number of *yes* answers here.

12–15: Excellent

8–11: Good

Fewer than 8: Reread Chapter 7, and make a plan for improving your mental and emotional health.

Chapter 8 Study Guide

> ## STUDY TIPS
> ✔ Read the chapter objectives.
> ✔ Look up any unfamiliar words.
> ✔ Read the questions below before you read the chapter.

As you read the chapter, answer the following questions. Later you can use this guide to review the information in the chapter.

Lesson 1

1. Define *communication*. List its requirements.

_____

_____

2. List and explain two types of communication.

_____

_____

3. Define *tact*.

_____

4. To avoid hurting other people's feelings, what question should you ask yourself before you speak?

_____

Lesson 2

5. List the different types of families that are common in the United States.

_____

6. List and briefly explain the ways in which families meet the needs of their members.

_____

_____

_____

_____

_____

7. List five common family challenges.

_____

8. List four ways to strengthen family relationships.

_____

_____

_____

Lesson 3

9. List the qualities found in a good friend.

_____

_____

10. Define *compromise*.

_____

11. What are *peers*, and what is *peer pressure?*

_____

_____

12. List two positive and two negative examples of peer pressure.

_____

Lesson 4

13. Explain *abstinence*.

_____

14. List four effective refusal skills.

_____

Activity 32 — Applying Health Skills

DeAnne's Diary

Read this entry from a teen's diary. Then answer the questions.

Dear Diary,

Today started off badly, but things got better. First thing this morning, Mom told me I had to come straight home to baby-sit. I guess I frowned because she said, "What is that look supposed to mean?" I told her that I was planning to stay late after school to work on my science project with Rick. We agreed that I could stay after school for an hour, and then come home to baby-sit.

I sat with Bev on the school bus. She was wearing this corny T-shirt—it says, "My mom went on vacation and all I got was this lousy shirt." Bev thinks it's a hoot. I think it makes her look silly. I told her it was cute, but that she looked much better in a sweater.

At school I found a note in my locker from Jenny. She wrote that the new guy in school, Antoine, was asking about me in the lunchroom. Great! He is so cute. I thought he was looking at me in math class later on, so I smiled. He smiled back! I'm going to have to get up the nerve to say hi to him one day.

Rick and I got a lot done after school. This evening we spent an hour on the phone going over what we still need to get done. He told me he is under a lot of time pressure, since he also plays in the band and works on weekends. I told Rick it must be really hard for him to get everything done. Well, I better get to sleep. It was a busy day—but a good one!

1. Name one example of verbal communication in DeAnne's diary.

_____

2. Give an example of nonverbal communication from the diary.

_____

3. Describe a use of body language from DeAnne's diary.

_____

4. Describe how DeAnne showed tact during her day.

_____

5. Name one example of empathy in the diary.

_____

Activity 33

Applying Health Skills

All in the Family

Imagine that you are at a family reunion. Your cousins share their family problems with you. On the lines below, write your advice.

Cousin Selena
"Things are going well in our family. Mom got a great promotion, and we're moving to a big city. Everyone is very excited—but I'm also a little nervous. After all, we've always lived in a small town. I'm not sure how I'll do in the city."
My advice is:

_____

_____

_____

Cousin Dan
"Dad is still looking for a job. It's weird. He used to be so full of energy. Now he doesn't even want to play basketball with me anymore. I don't show him how I feel, but seeing him this way makes me sad and angry at the same time."
My advice is:

_____

_____

Cousin Tanya
"I'm so worried. Mom and Dad have been fighting for months. Last week Dad moved out of the house. I think they may be fighting because they are disappointed with me. I don't know what to do."
My advice is:

_____

_____

Cousin Leroy
"Mom just hasn't been the same since her friend died. Why can't she cheer up? After all, it's been almost a year! She's sad because she thinks that no one is being understanding."
My advice is:

_____

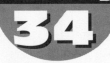

Activity 34

Applying Health Skills

Peer Pressure

Each statement below is a form of peer pressure. In the space to the left of each statement, write a plus sign (+) if it is positive peer pressure or a minus sign (−) if it is negative. Then, on the lines provided, describe the pressure and explain why it would or would not be a good idea to go along with the statement.

_____ 1. "Let's spray-paint our school colors all over town for School Spirit Week!"

_____

_____

_____ 2. "Want to go for a run? It'll help us get in shape for track season."

_____

_____

_____ 3. "You won't drink beer? How can you pass judgment if you won't even try it?"

_____

_____

_____

_____ 4. "Did you see the new kid in school? Let's trash his locker—we've got to show that we don't like his type around here."

_____

_____

_____ 5. "I think you should cut back on the hours you work after school and spend more time hitting the books—it will help you reach your goal of making the honor roll."

_____

_____

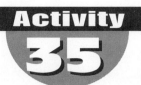

Applying Health Skills

Positive Pressure Statements

You can act as a positive influence on your peers. Read about each teen described below. On the lines that follow, write a positive pressure statement you could make to help the teen choose abstinence.

Charlie
Charlie is following in his older brother's footsteps as a star player on the school baseball team. Charlie's brother always chews tobacco when he plays. Charlie thinks that maybe he'll start chewing tobacco, too.

_____

Tiffany
Tiffany's boyfriend wants her to engage in sexual activity with him. He says all teens have sex. So far Tiffany has refused, but she doesn't want to lose him.

_____

Heather
This year, Heather is hanging out with the most popular crowd at school. A few of those students use alcohol and drugs. No one has pressured Heather to try alcohol and drugs yet, but one of her new friends is hosting a big party this weekend.

_____

Derek
Some boys at school have asked Derek if he wants to join their group. Derek wants to, since the boys seem so cool. Before he can join them, though, Derek must prove to the boys that he is "worthy" by shoplifting a CD from a music store at the mall.

_____

Brenda
Brenda's friends are all dating older teens. Brenda does not feel ready to date, but her friends are pressuring her to go out with them on group dates.

_____

Chapter 8 Health Inventory

How Is Your Social Health?

Read each statement below. Decide how it describes your social health habits. Write *always*, *sometimes*, or *never* in the space to the left of each statement.

_____ 1. When I give criticism, I try to praise the good points before pointing out weaknesses.

_____ 2. When pressured to do something dangerous or illegal, I rely on my values to make a decision.

_____ 3. I respect others' property.

_____ 4. I choose my friends carefully.

_____ 5. I am not afraid to ask adults I trust for advice.

_____ 6. I share my thoughts and feelings with members of my family.

_____ 7. I make an effort to spend quality time with my family.

_____ 8. I avoid interrupting others.

_____ 9. I make eye contact when speaking with others.

_____ 10. I show empathy when listening to others.

_____ 11. I think before I speak.

_____ 12. I use "I" messages to express myself.

_____ 13. I am aware of the messages I send with my body language.

_____ 14. I am willing to compromise to reach a solution that satisfies everyone.

_____ 15. I know and use the S.T.O.P. method of refusal.

Score yourself:

Give yourself 3 points for each *always* answer, 1 point for each *sometimes*, and 0 for each *never*. Write your score here.

36–45: You have excellent social health.

26–35: Your social health is good.

16–25: You can improve your social health.

Fewer than 16: Make a plan to build better relationships with your family, friends, and peers.

Chapter 9 Study Guide

As you read the chapter, answer the following questions. Later you can use this guide to review the information in the chapter.

Lesson 1

1. Define *conflict* and *prejudice*.

_____

_____

2. What are some of the most common reasons teens argue?

_____

_____

3. Give four suggestions for preventing serious conflicts.

_____

_____

Lesson 2

4. Define *nonviolent confrontation*.

_____

5. Explain how the *T.A.L.K. strategy* can help you remember how to negotiate by using the steps of conflict resolution.

_____

_____

6. Explain *mediation* and tell what quality the mediator must have.

_____

_____

Lesson 3

7. List four causes of violence.

_____

_____

8. Define *bully*.

_____

_____

9. List six things you should do and four you should not do if someone wants to fight.

_____

_____

_____

_____

_____

Lesson 4

10. What are the four major types of abuse?

_____

_____

11. What are four common reasons victims of abuse stay silent?

_____

_____

12. List three resources where someone who is dealing with abuse can find help.

_____

_____

Activity 36

Applying Health Skills

Stopping Conflicts

Write the missing term in each blank.

1. You may be able to stop a conflict from getting worse if you notice the warning signs that conflict may be escalating. List the "red flags":

   a. _____

   b. _____

   c. _____

   d. _____

   e. _____

   f. _____

   g. _____

   h. _____

   i. _____

2. Complete the following list of suggestions for preventing serious conflicts. Provide one example for each suggestion.

   • Practice good communication.

     Example: _____

     _____

   • Ignore some conflicts.

     Example: _____

     _____

   • Don't take sides.

     Example: _____

     _____

   • Show disapproval of fighting.

     Example: _____

     _____

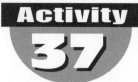

Activity 37 · Applying Health Skills

Resolving Conflicts

Write the missing term in each blank. Then answer the question.

neutral	mediation	mediator	negotiate	nonviolent confrontation

1. When Kenny sees two of his friends—a boy and a girl—arguing, he decides to stay _____, or promise not to take sides. They both call to him for support. How might Kenny help?

_____

2. Delores knows that _____, or resolving a conflict by peaceful methods, is better than fighting. What might she say to her peers to convince them to take this approach to deal with unavoidable conflicts?

_____

3. Bernard has been arguing with Jeremy. The boys have agreed to use _____ by using another person to help reach a solution that is acceptable to both sides. They choose Anthony to be the mediator. What quality must Anthony have if he is to be a good mediator?

_____

4. Sara and Sue are having a conflict. They decide to _____, or discuss their problems face-to-face in order to reach a solution. As they begin, each is thinking that someone must win and someone else must lose. What would be a better way for them to think of conflict resolution?

_____

_____

5. Louis and Sam have been in conflict for a while. They decide to ask Rocco to be a _____ to resolve their conflict. How can Rocco help resolve the conflict?

_____

Activity 38 Applying Health Skills

The Truth About Violence

Write *true* or *false* next to each statement below about violence in our society today.

_____ 1. Violence is a major public health problem in the United States.

_____ 2. People who commit violent acts often have learned to deal with their feelings, particularly anger, in healthful ways.

_____ 3. Prejudice is a factor that contributes to violence.

_____ 4. Teens are more than twice as likely as people in other age groups to be victims of violence.

_____ 5. To protect yourself, it is important to look like an easy target.

_____ 6. If someone wants to fight with you, you should be hostile, threatening, insulting, rude, or sarcastic.

_____ 7. People who are under the influence of alcohol or other drugs commit almost half of all violent crimes.

_____ 8. If you are wronged, you should try to even the score.

_____ 9. Some television programs may lead people to believe that violence is an acceptable way to settle disagreements.

_____ 10. A decline in moral values may not be a factor that has increased violence in our society.

_____ 11. The majority of teens are not violent and do not commit crimes.

_____ 12. Conflict resolution programs help teens to understand alternatives to violence.

_____ 13. Criminal gangs rarely have rules or symbols.

_____ 14. Some communities use Neighborhood Watch programs to make their neighborhoods safer.

_____ 15. Some schools use security cameras to help keep out weapons.

_____ 16. Schools are one place where young people do not have to worry about violence.

Activity 39 — Applying Health Skills

Identifying Abuse

Some people may think that reports of abuse are limited to physical problems. They may be unaware of the different kinds of abuse many people suffer. Read each news story below and answer the questions.

News Story 1

Police reported finding two young children in a home. Only a small amount of food was in the house, and the older child said that he had not seen their parents for several days.

1. What kind of abuse does the story illustrate?

_____

News Story 2

A judge issued a restraining order to prevent a woman's husband from entering her house. She claimed that he had beaten her once and had threatened to do so again.

2. What kind of abuse does the story illustrate?

_____

News Story 3

Friends of a runaway teen reported that he had often complained of being unable to live up to his family's standards. Some had been present to hear the family's constant criticism of his apparent underachievement in school.

3. What kind of abuse does the story imply?

_____

News Story 4

A teen girl reported that she had been touched and fondled against her will by a man who was a longtime friend of her family.

4. What kind of abuse does the story illustrate?

_____

Chapter 9 Health Inventory

Dealing with Conflict, Violence, and Abuse

Read the statements below. In the space at the left, write *yes* if the statement describes you or *no* if it does not describe you.

_____ 1. When I disagree with someone, I use "I" messages.

_____ 2. I am alert for the signs of anger in my body.

_____ 3. I can ignore conflicts about issues that are not worth my time and effort.

_____ 4. I avoid getting involved in conflicts between other people.

_____ 5. I know that a mediator must remain neutral to effectively assist people.

_____ 6. I believe that the key to breaking the cycle of abuse is to report it and talk about it.

_____ 7. I know that abuse is never the fault of the victim.

_____ 8. I believe that running away from home often leads to other problems.

_____ 9. I am aware of the warning signs of abuse.

_____ 10. If someone I know is being abused or is in danger of being abused, I know to seek help from a trusted adult.

_____ 11. I know about conflict resolution programs that help teens to understand alternatives to violence.

_____ 12. I know how to use refusal skills to avoid getting involved with gangs.

_____ 13. I know that alcohol and other drugs are factors that contribute to violence.

_____ 14. I know that the rise in crime may be related to easier access to weapons.

_____ 15. I accept others who are different from myself.

Score yourself:

Write the number of *yes* answers here.

12–15: You are well-informed about preventing violence and abuse.

8–11: You are beginning to get the message.

Fewer than 8: You still need to learn more about preventing violence and abuse.

Chapter 10 Study Guide

As you read the chapter, answer the following questions. Later you can use this guide to review the information in the chapter.

Lesson 1

1. List four risks associated with the use of smokeless tobacco.

_____

_____

2. Describe the harmful effect of tobacco on the nervous system.

_____

3. Describe the harmful effect of tobacco on the circulatory system.

_____

Lesson 2

4. List the parts of the respiratory system.

_____

5. List health problems of the respiratory system.

_____

6. List three simple tips to take good care of your respiratory system.

_____

_____

Lesson 3

7. Explain why people get "hooked" on tobacco products.

_____

_____

8. List and explain the two types of addiction.

_____

_____

_____

9. List six reasons teens use tobacco products.

_____

_____

_____

Lesson 4

10. Explain why sidestream smoke is harmful.

_____

_____

_____

11. Describe how a woman who uses tobacco during pregnancy seriously endangers the health of her unborn child.

_____

_____

_____

12. List two rights you have as a nonsmoker.

_____

_____

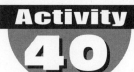

Activity 40

Use with Chapter 10, Lesson 1.

Applying Health Skills

What's in Tobacco Smoke?

Tobacco has harmful effects on almost all parts of the body. In the chart below, describe the dangerous substances that are found in tobacco smoke.

The Harmful Substances in Tobacco Smoke	
Nicotine	
Cyanide	
Methanol	
Carbon monoxide	
Tar	
Formaldehyde	

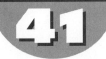

Activity 41 · Applying Health Skills

The Breathing Process

Fill in each blank with the correct term. Some terms are used more than once.

alveoli	carbon dioxide	inhaling	bronchi	diaphragm	exhaling
lungs	bronchioles	epiglottis	trachea	capillaries	

Stage One: _____

1. Your _____ moves down.

2. Air enters through the nose or mouth, then moves past the _____.

3. Air travels into the _____ and _____.

Stage Two: Inside the _____

4. The bronchi divide into smaller passages called _____.

5. Air passes into the _____, which are surrounded by _____.

6. _____ from the blood enters the _____.

Stage Three: _____

7. Your _____ pushes up, and your ribs move in and down, forcing air out of your _____.

8. The air, now containing _____, moves back through the bronchioles and bronchi, up the trachea, and out through the nose or mouth.

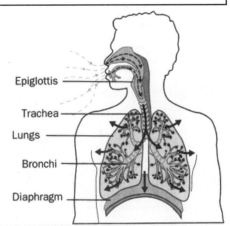

Epiglottis
Trachea
Lungs
Bronchi
Diaphragm

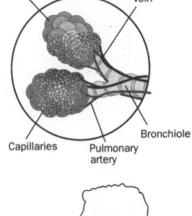

Alveoli
Pulmonary vein
Bronchiole
Capillaries
Pulmonary artery

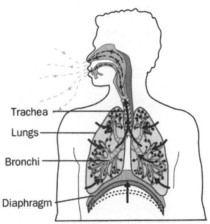

Trachea
Lungs
Bronchi
Diaphragm

Activity 42 — Applying Health Skills

Tobacco Addiction

Some smokers may not realize in what ways they are addicted to tobacco. Read the following statements. Then answer the questions that follow.

Sabrina's Phone Call
"I really can't talk on the phone unless I smoke a cigarette."

1. What type of addiction does this statement show?

_____

2. What is the reason for this effect?

_____

_____

Dan's Quick Exit
"I know I missed the most exciting part when I left the game last night, but I just had to go have a cigarette."

3. What type of addiction does this statement show?

_____

4. What is the reason for this effect?

_____

_____

Russell's Increasing Need
"I used to get by on half a pack of cigarettes a week, but lately, I don't feel right unless I smoke a lot more than that."

5. What aspect of physical dependence does this statement show?

_____

6. What is the reason for this effect?

_____

_____

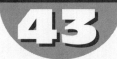

Activity 43   Applying Health Skills

Nonsmokers' Risks and Rights

Answer these questions about the risks that smoking places on nonsmokers and nonsmokers' rights.

1. Name two kinds of secondhand smoke that fill the air whenever someone smokes tobacco:

_____

_____

_____

_____

_____

2. Explain what passive smoking is and why it is harmful:

_____

_____

_____

_____

3. What are five benefits of being tobacco free?

_____

_____

_____

_____

4. What are two rights of nonsmokers?

_____

_____

_____

Chapter **10** Health Inventory

The Truth About Tobacco

Some of these statements about tobacco are facts, and some are myths. Identify each statement by writing *fact* or *myth* in the space at the left.

_____ 1. Smokeless tobacco is not as harmful and addictive as smoking.

_____ 2. Nicotine is as addictive as alcohol, cocaine, or heroin.

_____ 3. A single puff of tobacco smoke contains more than 4,000 chemicals.

_____ 4. Tobacco addiction is purely psychological.

_____ 5. Tobacco use reduces the flow of oxygen to the brain.

_____ 6. Secondhand smoke is not harmful to nonsmokers.

_____ 7. Tobacco use during pregnancy seriously endangers the health of the unborn child.

_____ 8. The government has banned smoking on all domestic airplane flights.

_____ 9. Carbon monoxide in tobacco smoke prevents the body from getting all the oxygen it needs.

_____ 10. Smoking for just a few years does not have negative effects.

_____ 11. Smokeless tobacco use can cause gum disease.

_____ 12. Tobacco use is linked to heart disease.

_____ 13. People who smoke cigars or pipes are more likely to develop cancers of the lip, mouth, and tongue.

_____ 14. The "cold turkey" method is the only effective way to quit tobacco use.

_____ 15. Tar in tobacco smoke forms a sticky coating on the tubes and air sacs inside the lungs.

Score yourself:

Give yourself 4 points for each correct answer.

48–60: Excellent—you really know the truth about tobacco.

32–44: Good—you are fairly well informed about tobacco.

Fewer than 32: Smoke is in your eyes! Learn the facts about tobacco.

Chapter Study Guide

STUDY TIPS

✔ Read the chapter objectives.

✔ Look up any unfamiliar words.

✔ Read the questions below before you read the chapter.

As you read the chapter, answer the following questions. Later you can use this guide to review the information in the chapter.

Lesson 1

1. Explain the difference between a *drug* and a *medicine.*

_____

_____

2. How are prescription medicines and over-the-counter (OTC) medicines different, and what do they have in common?

_____

_____

_____

Lesson 2

3. List the immediate effects and the long-term effects that alcohol has on the brain.

_____

_____

_____

4. List the parts of the body other than the brain that alcohol affects.

_____

Lesson 3

5. Describe the following types of drugs and list one general effect each can have on the body: marijuana, stimulants, and depressants.

_____

_____

_____

_____

6. Explain what *club drugs* are and why they are dangerous.

_____

_____

_____

Lesson 4

7. List and briefly describe the two main parts of the nervous system.

_____

_____

_____

_____

8. List the parts of the brain.

_____

Lesson 5

9. List six mental and emotional effects of the use of alcohol and drugs.

_____

_____

_____

_____

10. Explain why you need to be assertive to stay drug and alcohol free.

_____

_____

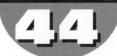

Applying Health Skills

Medicines and Drugs

Imagine that you are on a quiz show. One of the categories is drugs and medicines. The quiz show host presents only the answers. You must supply the questions.

1. **Answer:** A substance other than food that changes the structure or function of the body or mind

   Question: _____

2. **Answer:** A drug that prevents or cures illness or eases its symptoms

   Question: _____

3. **Answer:** Medicines that cause the immune system to produce substances that destroy specific germs before they can cause disease

   Question: _____

4. **Answer:** One type of medicine used to fight disease-causing germs

   Question: _____

5. **Answer:** A medicine that can be used safely only with a doctor's written permission

   Question: _____

6. **Answer:** Medicines that you can buy without a doctor's prescription

   Question: _____

7. **Answer:** Reactions to medicines other than the ones intended

   Question: _____

8. **Answer:** Only licensed pharmacists

   Question: _____

9. **Answer:** Read the label and take safety precautions

   Question: _____

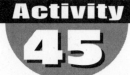

Activity 45   Use with Chapter 11, Lesson 2.

Applying Health Skills

Alcohol and Your Body

Alcohol has both short- and long-term effects on body systems. The diagram on this page shows the parts of the body that are affected by alcohol. On the lines below the diagram, identify each numbered body part and list one immediate effect and one long-term effect of alcohol on each body part.

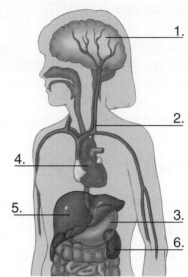

1. Body part: _____
 Immediate effect: _____
 Long-term effect: _____

2. Body part: _____
 Immediate effect: _____
 Long-term effect: _____

3. Body part: _____
 Immediate effect: _____
 Long-term effect: _____

4. Body part: _____
 Immediate effect: _____
 Long-term effect: _____

5. Body part: _____
 Immediate effect: _____
 Long-term effect: _____

6. Body part: _____
 Immediate effect: _____
 Long-term effect: _____

Activity 46 — Applying Health Skills

Commonly Abused Drugs

Listed below are five types of commonly abused drugs. Describe the main effect of each type of drug. Then, for each, list either two examples of the drug or one danger associated with its use.

1. Stimulants

Effect: _____

Examples: _____

2. Depressants

Effect: _____

Examples: _____

3. Narcotics

Effect: _____

Examples: _____

4. Hallucinogens

Effect: _____

Danger: _____

5. Inhalants

Effect: _____

Danger: _____

_____

Answer these questions.

6. Which type of drug do you think is the most dangerous? Why?

_____

7. Which type of drug do you think poses the greatest risk to teens? Why?

_____

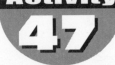

Activity 47

Applying Health Skills

The Body's Control System

Read the paragraph below. Fill in each blank with the appropriate term from the list below.

brain stem	motor neurons	cerebellum
cerebrum	sensory neurons	connecting neurons

Jared is sound asleep. His breathing is controlled by his

(**1**) _____. The alarm clock rings. (**2**) _____ in

Jared's ear receive information and send impulses to his brain. In Jared's

spinal cord and brain, (**3**) _____ translate the message of the

sound. As Jared wakes up, his (**4**) _____, the largest part of

his brain, interprets the sound. His brain sends a message to his arm mus-

cles along (**5**) _____. Jared's arm reaches out and turns off

the alarm. Jared gets out of bed and stands up, his balance maintained by

his (**6**) _____.

7. Write the numbers of the answers that are part of Jared's central nervous system.

   _____

8. Write the numbers of the answers that are part of Jared's peripheral nervous system.

   _____

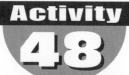

Applying Health Skills

Responsible Decisions

Read each situation below. In the space that follows, describe a responsible decision that each teen could make. Then, in the quotation marks, write what each teen could say to resolve the situation.

Situation 1
The "In" Crowd

Maria gets a phone call from her friend Cindy. Cindy says that they are invited to go to the movies with a popular group of kids. Maria knows that the group has a reputation for drinking. Maria doesn't want to drink. "Are you going to come along?" Cindy asks.

What should Maria do?

_____

_____

Situation 2
Stressed Out

Zak is against using drugs. He has the usual stress of homework, along with daily baseball practice and band practice twice a week. Now he also has to baby-sit this weekend. When Zak tells his friend Pete about his problems, Pete offers Zak some marijuana. "It will mellow you right out," Pete says.

What should Zak do?

_____

_____

Situation 3
Join the Team

Curt is proud to be on the football team. He respects the rules and follows them. The team captain invites Curt to come to his house to watch videos of their last game and have a few beers with the guys. "Are you on the team, or what?" the captain asks.

What should Curt do?

_____

_____

Chapter 11 Health Inventory

Alcohol, Drugs, and You

Here is a checklist about alcohol and drugs. In the space to the left, put a check (✔) next to each statement that describes you.

_____ 1. I know the short- and long-term effects of alcohol on body systems.

_____ 2. When I use an over-the-counter medicine, I read the label carefully.

_____ 3. I avoid social situations where substance use might take place.

_____ 4. I refuse to ride in a car driven by someone who has been drinking.

_____ 5. When I take a prescription drug, I follow the detailed instructions of the doctor and pharmacist.

_____ 6. I know effective refusal skills to help say no to drugs.

_____ 7. I realize that alcohol or drug abuse affect an abuser's family.

_____ 8. I know that teens who use substances are at risk for becoming victims of crime.

_____ 9. If I am in a place where someone is abusing drugs, I promptly leave.

_____ 10. I realize that people who are addicted to alcohol or drugs may try to hide the problem or deny that one exists.

_____ 11. I know that using alcohol or drugs will not help me relieve stress.

_____ 12. I never give my prescription medicines to others.

_____ 13. I am aware that alcoholism is an illness.

_____ 14. I know there are people and organizations I can turn to for help if I or someone I know has an alcohol or drug problem.

_____ 15. I don't give in to feelings of low self-esteem.

Score yourself:

Write the number of checks here.

12–15: You know the facts about alcohol and drug abuse.

8–11: You know something about substance abuse, but you should know more.

Fewer than 8: You're kidding yourself about alcohol and drugs. Read Chapter 11 again and find out the facts.

Chapter 12 Study Guide

As you read the chapter, answer the following questions. Later you can use this guide to review the information in the chapter.

Lesson 1

1. What are *communicable diseases*, and what causes them?

_____

_____

_____

2. List four types of pathogens.

_____

_____

Lesson 2

3. List the five major barriers against pathogens.

_____

4. What is the *immune system?*

_____

_____

5. List two ways your body builds immunity.

_____

_____

Lesson 3

6. List six communicable diseases.

_____

_____

7. Explain how the three most common types of hepatitis can be contracted.

_____

_____

_____

Lesson 4

8. What are *sexually transmitted infections (STIs)?* List five common STIs.

_____

_____

9. List the ways in which HIV is almost always spread.

_____

_____

_____

10. What is the only sure way to protect yourself against unintended pregnancy and STIs?

_____

Lesson 5

11. List four guidelines that you should follow to protect yourself from pathogens.

_____

_____

_____

_____

_____

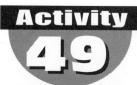

Activity 49

Applying Health Skills

Danger! Disease!

Use this page as your personal warning poster about the pathogens that cause communicable diseases. Fill in the blanks below.

Pathogen: _____

Description: The smallest and simplest disease-causing organisms.

Diseases they cause (name 10):

_____

_____

Pathogen: _____

Description: Tiny one-celled organisms that live nearly everywhere.

Diseases they cause (name 5):

_____

_____

Pathogen: _____

Description: Primitive life-forms, such as molds or yeasts, that cannot make their own food.

Diseases they cause:

_____

_____

Pathogen: _____

Description: One-celled organisms that have a more complex structure than bacteria.

Diseases they cause:

_____

_____

Activity 50 — Applying Health Skills

Use with Chapter 12, Lesson 2.

Defending Your Body

Complete the chart below. In the second column, write *MB* if the defense is part of your body's five major barriers, *NS* if it is a non-specific response of your immune system, or *S* if it is a specific response. Then, in the third column, describe the immediate result of the defense.

Defense	Type of Defense	Result
Mucous membranes that line the nose and throat trap pathogens.	_____	
Phagocytes release a special protein called interferon.	_____	
Your body reacts to antigens by producing antibodies.	_____	
T cells identify an antigen as an invader.	_____	
You develop a fever.	_____	
When a foreign object gets into your eye, tears develop.	_____	
Special white cells called phagocytes attack the invading pathogens.	_____	

List two ways in which your body builds immunity.

1. _____

2. _____

Activity 51 — Applying Health Skills

You're the Doctor

Read each case below. Then, for each case, diagnose the disease, name its cause, and recommend treatment.

Case 1

A teacher has a fever, cough, weakness, chills, and is having difficulty breathing.

Disease: _____

Cause: _____

Recommendation: _____

_____

Case 2

This teen has swollen lymph nodes in the neck and throat, is often very tired, has no appetite, and has a fever, headache, and a sore throat.

Disease: _____

Cause: _____

Recommendation: _____

_____

Case 3

A woman's skin has turned yellowish. She is weak, nauseated, and has a fever, headache, sore throat, and not much appetite.

Disease: _____

Cause: _____

Recommendation: _____

_____

Case 4

A boy has a red and painful throat, fever, swollen and tender lymph nodes in the neck, and a headache.

Disease: _____

Cause: _____

Recommendation: _____

_____

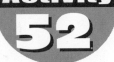

Activity 52   Use with Chapter 12, Lesson 4.

Applying Health Skills

Set Them Straight

Each teen quoted below has misconceptions about sexually transmitted infections. In each case, set the teen straight by writing a fact about STIs on the lines after the quote.

Mark
"If I get an STI, I'll just go to the doctor for a shot. That'll take care of me."

_____

_____

Janine
"My boyfriend had an STI, but the symptoms went away, so I'm in no danger of catching it from him."

_____

_____

Karen
"My neighbor has AIDS. I'll never go near a swimming pool after he's been in it!"

_____

_____

Jamal
"I'm never going to donate blood again—I might get HIV."

_____

_____

Hector
"I don't have to worry about STIs as long as I only have sexual contact with a few people."

_____

_____

Activity 53

Applying Health Skills

Spread the Word—Not the Germ

Imagine that you are planning a public awareness campaign to stop the spread of communicable diseases. Create signs to post at each of the places listed below. Make signs that tell how to avoid spreading pathogens at each specific place.

Sign #1: Near the Bathroom Sink

Sign #2: In the School Cafeteria

Sign #3: On a Hiking Trail in the Woods

Sign #4: In Your Kitchen at Home

Chapter **12** Health Inventory

Stopping Communicable Diseases

Read the following checklist of habits that will help you stop the spread of communicable diseases. In the space to the left of each, place a check (✔) if you have that habit.

_____ 1. I cover my mouth and nose with a tissue when I cough or sneeze.

_____ 2. I wash my hands before handling or eating food.

_____ 3. I take proper precautions and wear adequate clothing when I hike through habitats where there may be ticks.

_____ 4. When I am ill, I stay home and avoid close contact with other people.

_____ 5. I eat plenty of fruits, vegetables, and whole-grain breads.

_____ 6. I abstain from sexual activity.

_____ 7. I participate in regular physical activity.

_____ 8. I do not share eating utensils, dishes, glasses, bottles, cans, or food with others.

_____ 9. I keep my hands away from my mouth, nose, and eyes.

_____ 10. I scrub under my fingernails when I wash my hands.

_____ 11. When I take a prescribed medication, I follow the directions and my doctor's orders carefully.

_____ 12. I get medical treatment if I need it.

_____ 13. I know how to manage stress.

_____ 14. I encourage other people to follow wise health practices.

_____ 15. I bathe or shower daily.

Score yourself:

Write the number of checks here.

12–15: Congratulations! You're likely to stay healthy and fit.

8–11: Your health habits are fair, but they could be improved.

Fewer than 8: You're in danger! Read Chapter 12 again—and change your habits.

Chapter 13 Study Guide

As you read the chapter, answer the following questions. Later you can use this guide to review the information in the chapter.

Lesson 1

1. What is a *noncommunicable disease?*

_____

2. What are four categories of noncommunicable diseases, based on their causes?

_____

_____

3. What are *histamines?*

_____

4. What is *asthma?*

_____

_____

Lesson 2

5. What is a *tumor?* Explain the two types of tumors.

_____

_____

6. List the four most common types of cancer.

_____

7. What are three ways cancer is treated?

_____

8. What can you do to help lower your risk of certain cancers?

_____

Lesson 3

9. Define each of the following types of heart disease: *arteriosclerosis, atherosclerosis, heart attack.* Define the following related disorders and conditions: *hypertension, stroke.*

_____

_____

_____

_____

_____

_____

10. List the possible treatments for heart disease.

_____

Lesson 4

11. What are *diabetes* and *insulin?* How are they related?

_____

_____

_____

12. What is *arthritis?*

_____

13. Compare the two main types of arthritis.

_____

_____

_____

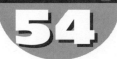

Activity 54   Use with Chapter 13, Lesson 1.

Applying Health Skills

Allergies and Asthma

Fill in the blanks.

Allergens

List six common allergens and one common source for that allergen.

1. _____

    Source: _____

2. _____

    Source: _____

3. _____

    Source: _____

4. _____

    Source: _____

5. _____

    Source: _____

6. _____

    Source: _____

Allergic Reactions

List two allergic reactions involving each body part or system.

Eyes _____

Nose _____

Throat _____

Skin _____

Respiratory System _____

Digestive System _____

Asthma Triggers

List four common asthma triggers.

_____

Activity 55 — Applying Health Skills

Understanding Cancer

Complete the chart, using the information from Figure 13.5 on page 371 of your textbook.

Forms of Cancer

Form of Cancer	Risk Factors	Important Fact
Breast cancer	Family history, more common in women over age 50, but can also occur in younger women and in men	
Reproductive cancers		
colon and rectum cancer		
Leukemia		
Lung cancer		
Lymphoma		
Skin cancer		

Activity 56 — Applying Health Skills

Understanding Heart Disease

Each patient listed below is being treated for heart disease. In each case, write the missing term in the space to the left of the case study.

angioplasty	atherosclerosis	hypertension
arteriosclerosis	heart attack	pacemaker

Case Studies

1. Patient A is undergoing _____, a surgical procedure in which an instrument with a tiny balloon attached is inserted into an artery to clear a blockage.

2. Medication helps Patient B handle her _____, or high blood pressure.

3. Patient C suffered a _____ when the blood supply to his heart slowed or stopped and his heart muscle was damaged.

4. Bypass surgery helped Patient D overcome _____, in which fatty substances built up on the inner lining of his arteries.

5. _____, a thickening and hardening of the arteries, puts Patient E at risk of stroke.

6. Patient F uses a _____, an electronic device that helps the heart to beat regularly.

Do you know how to prevent heart disease? Next to each factor, write a plus (1) sign if it can help keep your heart healthy. Write a minus (2) sign if it can increase the risk of developing heart disease.

_____ 7. A high intake of saturated fats.

_____ 8. Cigarette smoking.

_____ 9. Regular physical activity.

_____ 10. Eating fruits and vegetables daily.

_____ 11. Unmanaged stress.

_____ 12. Maintaining a healthy weight.

Activity 57
Applying Health Skills

Diabetes and Arthritis

Identify each term in the column on the right by matching it with the correct description in the column on the left. Write the letter of the term in the space provided.

_____ 1. A hormone that regulates the level of glucose in the blood.

_____ 2. The more common type of diabetes.

_____ 3. The type of diabetes that usually develops during childhood or adolescence.

_____ 4. Affects about 43 million people in the United States.

_____ 5. The more common type of arthritis.

_____ 6. A disease that prevents the body from converting food into energy.

_____ 7. The most serious and disabling form of arthritis.

a. type 2
b. arthritis
c. diabetes
d. insulin
e. osteoarthritis
f. rheumatoid arthritis
g. type 1

Answer the following questions about diabetes and arthritis. Write your answers on the lines provided.

8. What are some ways to manage diabetes?

_____

9. Explain the difference between type 1 and type 2 diabetes in relation to insulin.

_____

_____

10. Explain the difference between osteoarthritis and rheumatoid arthritis in relation to the joints usually affected.

_____

_____

_____

Chapter **13** Health Inventory

Avoiding Noncommunicable Diseases

Read each statement below. Decide whether it describes your health behavior. Write *always*, *sometimes*, or *never* in the space to the left of each statement.

_____ **1.** I avoid alcoholic beverages.

_____ **2.** I limit the amount of fat I eat.

_____ **3.** I manage stress in healthful ways.

_____ **4.** I participate in physical activity each day.

_____ **5.** I avoid tobacco in any form.

_____ **6.** I limit my intake of salt.

_____ **7.** I eat 3–5 servings of fruits and vegetables each day.

_____ **8.** I avoid being in the sun between 10 a.m. and 4 p.m.

_____ **9.** I get regular medical checkups.

_____ **10.** I choose low-fat snacks.

_____ **11.** I include plenty of whole grains in my diet.

_____ **12.** I maintain a healthy weight.

_____ **13.** I limit eating grilled foods.

_____ **14.** I regularly look for changes in moles on my skin.

_____ **15.** I check for the seven warning signs of cancer.

Score yourself:

Give yourself 3 points for each *always* answer, 1 point for each *sometimes*, and 0 for each *never.* Write your score here.

36–45: You are doing an excellent job of avoiding disease.

26–35: You take fairly good care of your body.

16–25: Be careful not to develop a lifestyle that could lead to disease.

Fewer than 16: Reread Chapter 13, and make a plan for changing your habits.

Chapter **14** Study Guide

As you read the chapter, answer the following questions. Later you can use this guide to review the information in the chapter.

Lesson 1

1. What does it mean to be safety conscious?

_____

_____

_____

2. What is an accident chain? What are three ways to break an accident chain?

_____

_____

_____

Lesson 2

3. What are some of the leading causes of fires in the home?

_____

_____

4. List the rules that can help you prevent poisonings.

_____

_____

_____

Lesson 3

5. What are three tips that will help you stay safe in your neighborhood and reduce your chances of becoming a victim?

_____

6. What are the common-sense rules for recreational safety?

_____

Lesson 4

7. What are weather emergencies? What are the most common weather emergencies?

_____

_____

8. List the safety rules to follow in any flood situation.

_____

_____

_____

9. How do *earthquakes* and *aftershocks* differ?

_____

_____

Lesson 5

10. Define *abdominal thrust*s and *chest thrusts*.

_____

_____

_____

11. List the three methods to stop or slow blood loss.

_____

_____

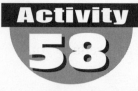

Activity 58

Use with Chapter 14, Lesson 1.

Applying Health Skills

The Accident Chain

Here are two examples of accident chains. Rewrite each step in each chain in such a way that the accident would be avoided.

	Timmy	Janelle
Situation	Timmy agreed to study with his friends, but now he is running late.	Janelle is taking down holiday decorations by herself.
Unsafe Habit	Timmy gets on his bike without tucking his pant legs into his socks.	Janelle does not have the proper tools for the job.
Unsafe Action	Timmy bicycles as fast as he can to the library.	Janelle uses a screwdriver to pry out nails.
Accident	Timmy's pant leg gets caught in his bicycle chain. He falls from his bike.	The screwdriver slips and slices into Janelle's hand.
Result	Timmy's bike is damaged. He scrapes his arm and sprains his wrist.	Janelle has a bad cut on her hand.

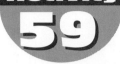

Activity 59 — Applying Health Skills

Who Is Safest?

Joanna and Betsy are checking their homes for safety hazards. Look at each list. Place a (✔) check next to each safety hazard.

Joanna's Home

_____   Smoke alarms outside each bedroom door.

_____   Cleaning fluids stored in an unlocked cabinet under sink.

_____   Rugs secured with tape.

_____   Electrical extension cord taped down beneath carpet.

_____   Loaded gun stored in drawer near parents' bed.

_____   Stereo, TV, and VCR all plugged into same wall outlet.

Betsy's Home

_____   Fire extinguisher in kitchen.

_____   Hair dryer, with frayed cord, is plugged into outlet.

_____   Well-lighted stairways free of loose objects.

_____   Paint cans and old rags stored in hall closet near a heating vent.

_____   Folding gates at top and bottom of staircase.

_____   Medicine stored in a kitchen dish cabinet.

Count the number of checks in each column. Write those numbers here:

Joanna's home: _____   Betsy's home: _____

On the lines that follow, write three things that one of the girls could do to make her home safer.

_____

_____

_____

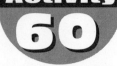

Applying Health Skills

Activity 60

Safety Sound Bites

Read each suggestion or comment below. On the line that follows, write a response that would help keep the speaker safe and sound.

1. "Let's race to the end of the dock and dive into the lake."

_____

_____

2. "Only babies wear bicycle helmets."

_____

_____

3. "This ski slope is a little steeper than I'm used to, but I'll sure look cool when I ski down it."

_____

_____

4. "Oops! The light just turned yellow—but if we run, we can make it across the street."

_____

5. "On the way home from the movie tonight, let's take a shortcut through the alley."

_____

_____

6. "Swimming is a great workout—but no one wants to swim with me. I think I'll just take a dip in the lake by myself."

_____

_____

7. "The sky is really getting dark, but the storm's not supposed to come until tonight, so we can still get in our hike."

_____

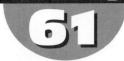

Activity 61

Use with Chapter 14, Lesson 4.

Applying Health Skills

Warning!

Read the situations below. On the lines following each situation, write what you would do to remain safe.

Situation 1
You are riding in a car on a dark, stormy day. An announcer on the radio states that a tornado warning has been declared in your county. You see a dark, funnel-shaped cloud in the distance.

_____

_____

_____

Situation 2
You are at home watching TV during a driving rainstorm. An emergency bulletin interrupts the program to announce that there is a flood watch for your town.

_____

_____

_____

Situation 3
At home, you have just used your computer to log on to the Internet. You check the news and learn that your state is being battered by thunderstorms. You hear thunder rumble outside.

_____

_____

_____

Situation 4
You are listening to the radio as you wash your bicycle and some outdoor furniture near the garage. You hear an announcer report that a hurricane is heading your way.

_____

_____

_____

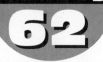

Applying Health Skills

First Aid

Identify each term in the column on the right by matching it with the correct description in the column on the left. Write the letter of the term in the space provided.

_____ 1. A first aid procedure in which someone forces air into the lungs of a person who is not breathing.

_____ 2. Should be given only by specially trained individuals.

_____ 3. Use this on an infant or small child who is choking.

_____ 4. Marked by the skin turning red.

_____ 5. The procedure to save an adult from choking.

_____ 6. Marked by blisters in the affected area.

a. abdominal thrusts

b. cardiopulmonary resuscitation

c. chest thrusts

d. first-degree burn

e. rescue breathing

f. second-degree burn

Answer the following questions about first aid. Write your answers on the lines provided.

7. Define CPR. Briefly explain the first steps, or ABCs, of CPR.

_____

_____

_____

_____

8. Explain the differences between first aid procedures for adults and infants who are choking.

_____

_____

_____

Chapter 14 Health Inventory

Crisis Management

Do you know the rules for dealing with an emergency? In the space at the left, put a check (✔) next to each statement that describes you or your home.

_____ **1.** I am aware that safety is important, and I am careful to act in a safe manner.

_____ **2.** In my house, all medicines have child-resistant caps.

_____ **3.** I wear a helmet when bicycling, skating, skateboarding, or riding a scooter.

_____ **4.** I never use an electrical appliance near water or if I am wet.

_____ **5.** The stove in our house is kept clean.

_____ **6.** I know basic first aid techniques.

_____ **7.** There is an emergency supplies kit in my house.

_____ **8.** I take a buddy when I go hiking.

_____ **9.** I obey traffic regulations when bicycling.

_____ **10.** As a pedestrian, I never assume that motorists will obey the law.

_____ **11.** There is a fire extinguisher in my home.

_____ **12.** In my home the smoke alarms are tested once a month.

_____ **13.** I use a step stool to get items that are out of reach.

_____ **14.** I do not overload electrical outlets.

_____ **15.** My family and I have an escape plan in case of fire.

Score yourself:

Write the number of checks here.

12–15: You're safe at home!—and away from home, too.

8–11: You need to be more careful.

Fewer than 8: Accidents and emergencies can happen to anyone. Reread Chapter 14 so that you are prepared.

Chapter **15** Study Guide

STUDY TIPS

✔ Read the chapter objectives.

✔ Look up any unfamiliar words.

✔ Read the questions below before you read the chapter.

   As you read the chapter, answer the following questions. Later you can use this guide to review the information in the chapter.

Lesson 1

1. Where does most air pollution come from?

_____

_____

_____

2. What happens when fossil fuels burn? What are two products that result?

_____

_____

_____

3. Define *ozone.* Explain how ozone can be both helpful and harmful.

_____

_____

_____

4. Name the two sources of the water that people drink, and explain or give an example of each.

_____

_____

_____

Lesson 2

5. For what does the acronym *EPA* stand? What is the EPA and what does it do?

_____

_____

_____

6. For what does the acronym *OSHA* stand? What is OSHA and what does it do?

_____

_____

_____

7. List four ways that people can reduce air pollution.

_____

_____

_____

8. List four ways that people can prevent water pollution.

_____

_____

_____

9. What are the Three Rs that you can use to keep garbage out of landfills?

_____

_____

10. List five types of common household items that can be recycled.

_____

_____

11. What is one way to conserve energy while cooking?

_____

_____

Activity 63   Applying Health Skills

Pollution Words

Define the words as indicated and answer the related questions.

1. What is the difference between *biodegradable* and *nonbiodegradable* materials? List an example of each.

_____

_____

_____

_____

2. Define *hazardous wastes* and list four examples.

_____

_____

_____

3. What are *acid rain* and *smog?* What is the source of both?

_____

_____

4. What is *ozone?* What is its source?

_____

_____

5. What is the difference between *surface water* and *groundwater?* Why are oil spills and chemical waste a threat to these sources of water?

_____

_____

_____

Activity 64

Applying Health Skills

Reduce, Reuse, Recycle

Suggest a way to reduce, reuse, or recycle each waste item listed below. Then answer the question that follows. One item has been filled in as an example.

Waste Item	Reduce	Reuse	Recycle
paper grocery bag	Use your own basket or cloth bags instead of paper.	Carry groceries again.	Use for crafts projects.
glass tomato sauce jar			
stack of used computer printer paper			
out-of-fashion jeans			
used juice boxes			

Based on your suggestions, which types of products would you say are the worst for the environment? Explain.

_____

_____

_____

_____

_____

_____

_____

_____

Chapter **15** Health Inventory

Health

Do you take steps to protect yourself and the environment from the health hazards of pollution? In the space at the left, put a check (✔) next to each statement that describes you or your home.

_____ 1. I carpool or take public transportation when I can.

_____ 2. I ride my bike or walk to nearby activities.

_____ 3. I remain tobacco free.

_____ 4. In my home we use biodegradable soaps, detergents, and bleaches.

_____ 5. I do not throw hazardous materials out with the regular trash.

_____ 6. I clean up after my pets.

_____ 7. I don't litter.

_____ 8. In my home, we accumulate a full load before we wash laundry or run the dishwasher.

_____ 9. I turn off the television when it's not in use.

_____ 10. I pick up litter left by others.

_____ 11. I recycle aluminum, cardboard, glass, paper, and plastic.

_____ 12. I avoid using disposable plates and cups.

_____ 13. During cold weather, I wear an extra layer of clothing instead of turning up the thermostat.

_____ 14. I switch off the lights when I leave a room.

_____ 15. When cooking a small amount of food, I use a microwave or toaster oven instead of a conventional oven.

Score yourself:

Write the number of checks here.

12–15: You're acting responsibly toward the environment.

8–11: You could do more to reduce pollution.

Fewer than 8: The environment is everyone's responsibility. Reread Chapter 15 to review the steps you can take.

Notes

Notes

Notes

Notes

Notes

Notes